CHRONIC RADIATION HAZARDS

An Experimental Study with Fast Neutrons

CHRONIC RADIATION HAZARDS

An Experimental Study with Fast Neutrons

by

G. J. NEARY, R. J. MUNSON
and R. H. MOLE

Medical Research Council Radiobiological Research Unit, Atomic Energy Research Establishment, Harwell

PERGAMON PRESS

NEW YORK · LONDON
LOS ANGELES · PARIS

1957

PUBLISHED BY
PERGAMON PRESS

122 East 55th Street, New York 22, N.Y.
4 & 5 Fitzroy Square, London W.1.
24 Rue des Écoles, Paris Ve
10638, South Wilton Place, Los Angeles 47, California

Library of Congress Card Number 57-14862

CONTENTS

PREFACE

THERE is an increasingly widespread interest in environmental hazards from chronic exposure to all kinds of potentially toxic agents, not only radiations and radioactive materials but also chemicals of every description. The interest is no longer confined to purely occupational hazards, in fact it is often heightened by the realization that the agent may affect everyone in a population, e.g. agene in the manufacture of bread. There is also a widespread feeling that possibly toxic materials should be tested by animal experiment before human beings are exposed to them.

This monograph describes in some detail a large-scale chronic experiment on one particular kind of environmental hazard, namely ionizing radiation. Besides their specialized interest, the results may show what sort of information on chronic toxicity may be gained by animal experimentation. The deficiencies may well be more valuable, for there is no general agreement about the limits of usefulness of such experiments. The general question of how far the results of chronic toxicity experiments are in fact applicable to human problems is a most important one. Discussion is hampered by a shortage of relevant facts but radiation toxicity should provide a useful basis for discussion since human and animal experience are both becoming available.

The work described here is in one sense unique, since throughout nearly six years the daily running of a nuclear reactor was adjusted to the needs of a biological experiment. Nevertheless, however laborious the work involved in arranging the radiation exposures to the animals, it is easier from the biological point of view to carry out a chronic toxicity experiment with penetrating radiation than with any chemical toxic agent. The radiation may be administered without handling the animals or modifying their food or drink, and it can be relied upon to penetrate the further recesses of the body without being affected by the permeability barriers and metabolic side-tracks which modify the action of every chemical agent however it be administered.

ACKNOWLEDGEMENTS

AN investigation of the biological effects of chronic neutron irradiation was suggested by Sir John Cockcroft, Director of the Atomic Energy Research Establishment, and Professor J. S. Mitchell, Consultant to the Establishment. The experiment was carried out with the encouragement and assistance of Dr. J. F. Loutit, Director of the Medical Research Council Radiobiological Research Unit at A.E.R.E. The irradiation facilities on GLEEP could not have been constructed or used without the active co-operation and forbearance of Dr. J. V. Dunworth, Head of the Reactor Physics Division, and of Mr. F. C. Colmer and Mr. E. Lockett, successively Chief Operating Engineers of GLEEP, 1950–1955.

Mr. B. G. Chapman and Mrs. M. E. J. Young, formerly members of the scientific staff of the M.R.C. Unit, assisted greatly in the experimental work involved in the preparation of the irradiation tanks, with technical help from Mr. C. F. Wright and other members of the Unit's workshop. Mr. A. Palmer and Mr. J. East and other members of the animal house staff raised the stocks of mice and were responsible for their care throughout the experiment. Mr. D. Stock and Mr. S. Weal were responsible for the technical supervision of the irradiation from day to day, and for keeping records of exposure and dosage. The computations for the statistical analysis of the results were carried out by Miss J. Perrett. The preparation of pathological specimens was done by Mr. J. Wyatt, and much of the work devoted to determining r.b.e.'s by Mr. G. Jeffreys and Miss C. Dempsey.

Some further acknowledgements are made at the appropriate places in the text; in addition, there were many other of our colleagues at Harwell, too numerous to mention individually, who contributed in a variety of ways during this experiment.

We are grateful to Mr. R. M. Manwaring, Librarian, M.R.C. Unit, for preparation of the Index.

CHAPTER I

EXPERIMENTAL DESIGN

1. INTRODUCTION

FAST neutrons may be an environmental hazard around nuclear reactors and some machines for accelerating particles, and it is therefore of practical as well as academic importance to get some idea of the likely ill-effects of chronic irradiation by fast neutrons. There are only fragmentary data on man and evidence from animal experiments is scanty. Qualitatively, one would expect the ill-effects to be similar to those produced by chronic irradiation with other forms of ionizing radiation. Quantitatively, it is well known that the dose required to produce any given effect differs for different kinds of radiation and that the magnitude of this difference depends on the particular biological effect examined. This report describes an experiment planned to obtain a better appreciation of the hazards to be expected from low and very low levels of chronic irradiation by fast neutrons.

The neutron sources for earlier work of this sort were of two kinds, a pile (Henshaw, Snider, Riley, Stapleton and Zirkle, 1946; and Henshaw, Riley and Stapleton, 1947), and cyclotrons (Biochemical Research Foundation, 1947; Evans, 1948, 1949; Ely, Ross, Metcalfe, Inda, Barnett and Casarett, 1954). From the results of these and other experiments it has been suggested that the relative effects of small daily doses of fast neutrons as compared with gamma rays could become more pronounced the longer the duration of the exposure (for summary of evidence see Mitchell, 1952). However, in none of these earlier experiments was irradiation continued beyond ninety weeks, and the greater part of the work was on animals exposed and observed for less than a year and at dose rates of the order of 15 rads weekly and more. Moreover, the experimental techniques introduced two disadvantages, in that the daily irradiations were concentrated into a small fraction only of the day, and involved additional handling and disturbance of the animals every day when presenting them to the source of neutrons. There were thus good reasons for a new experiment permitting continuous exposure of animals throughout their lives and including dose rates near to the 'maximum permissible' dose rate for human exposure. Furthermore, it was desirable that the neutron doses should be measured in terms of energy deposition in tissue (reps or rads) instead of the previously employed 'n' or 'N' units.

At the outset it was necessary to choose some index of chronic radiation damage. Earlier experiments on the effects of daily irradiation by gamma rays (Lorenz, Heston, Eschenbrenner and Deringer, 1947) and by fast neutrons (Evans, 1948; Henshaw *et al.*, 1947) suggested that shortening of the life span was more sensitive than change in the blood picture, loss of weight or tumour production, and was certainly easier to measure, since there need be no observational error in deciding the day of death. The effect of radiation would then be measured by the excess of deaths in an irradiated group over those occurring in another control group of animals identical with the irradiated group in all respects save the irradiation. At low dose rates the excess of deaths would be small, and might not be appreciable until a large proportion of the animals in both groups had died. A small excess mortality can only be detected with large numbers of animals, and a figure of about one hundred per group was judged to be desirable, which meant in practice that mice were the only animals which could be used.

Mice usually live for more than two years under laboratory conditions and the only reliable source of daily irradiation by fast neutrons for such a prolonged period was a nuclear reactor. The fast neutrons produced within a reactor are too heavily contaminated with slow neutrons and gamma rays to be useful. However, fast neutrons sufficiently free from other radiations could be obtained from the thermal neutrons of the reactor by utilizing the fission reaction in uranium suitably arranged outside the reactor. The Harwell graphite pile GLEEP was suitable for this purpose. Four large holes in the upper face of the concrete pile shield were uncovered and uranium was inserted in the gaps, followed by slow neutron and gamma ray absorbers (see Chap. I, § 8, p. 10 and Fig. 2). A sensibly uniform flux of fast neutrons was obtained in each of four areas, 4¼ ft. square, and this large space allowed 100 mice to be housed in each area without overcrowding. The animals lived out their lives in ordinary animal cages, undisturbed except for the routine of animal care (Fig. 3).

With four independent exposure areas available it was possible to choose three different dose rates of fast neutrons while keeping the fourth area for a control group of animals which was to receive the same level of unavoidable gamma radiation as the other three (Chap. I, §9 (iv), p. 19). A fifth group of animals was kept free from irradiation other than natural background. The three neutron dose rates were chosen after consideration of the best information available on the effect on mice of chronic gamma irradiation (Lorenz *et al.*, 1947) and on the possible extreme values for the relative biological efficiency (r.b.e.) of fast neutrons as compared with gamma rays (see Chap. I, §3, p. 4). In addition to the main experiment on reduction of life span, some shorter-term neutron and gamma irradiations were carried out to determine directly the relative biological efficiencies for a variety of other effects. A direct determination of the r.b.e. for shortening of life span was not possible since long-term concurrent gamma irradiation of similar groups of animals was not practicable at that time. An experiment of this kind was begun in 1954, and will be reported later.

An alternative method of using a reactor for irradiation of animals with fast neutrons was that of Henshaw *et al.* (1946, 1947). These workers constructed a trolley to carry the animals and their surrounding uranium through a tunnel into the thermal neutron flux inside the pile shield and back again. Similar tunnels were available in the larger Harwell graphite pile BEPO but there were strong biological reasons against using them. It seemed unlikely that reliable results could be obtained from an experiment in which animals had to be loaded daily into special irradiation cages and subjected to noise and a thermally hot environment which it would be difficult to ventilate. It would have been impossible to ensure that the control animals were frightened as much and mechanically damaged as much as the irradiated animals. Moreover, the irradiation would have lasted but a few minutes daily, and large and unforeseeable variations were to be expected in the operation of this pile.

2. CHOICE OF ANIMAL

A mouse strain with a naturally high incidence of tumours or malignant disease was one to avoid, since the main purpose of the experiment was to detect a shortening of life span. At the same time it was desirable to use an inbred strain in order to reduce the natural variability of life span, and a vigorous, long-lived strain since it was possible that the longer the duration of the experiment the smaller the dose rate which would produce a detectable effect. Our existing mouse colony included CBA mice obtained from Dr. T. C. Carter, then at The Institute of Animal Genetics, Edinburgh, and by him from the animal stocks of the British Empire Cancer Campaign laboratories. The CBA mice in our laboratory all stemmed from an original breeding trio, and had been bred at first by sib-mating and subsequently by inbreeding within the laboratory. They had proved very consistent in their response to single doses of X rays and since they met all the other requirements were chosen for this experiment.

In order to get a uniform experimental stock of sufficient size to fill all five tanks the following breeding plan was adopted. From a common pair of ancestors, breeding lines had been developed by matings between brothers and sisters exclusively. After five or six generations matings were set up between half-sibs or cousins from ten different breeding lines. Their first litters were divided into five groups, each group containing two sets of litters, one from each of the original half-sib or cousin matings. On 8 September 1950 the males of one set of litters were placed with the females of the other and conversely, within each group. The experimental mice were obtained from the first litters of this second series of matings.

These litters were sorted according to date of birth, series I of forty litters born 28 and 29 September 1950, series II of thirty-eight litters born from 30 September to 2 October 1950, and series III of twenty-five litters born from 4 to 12 October 1950. A number of empty mouse cages was placed in a row, three for every five litters, and the four male mice from the first litter of series I were put one in each of the first four cages. Then the three male mice from the next litter were put one into each of the next three cages and so on, till there was one mouse in each cage. Then a second mouse was put into each of the cages in turn and so on, until all the series I males had been caged in groups of five. The same procedure was carried out for the females of series I and for the males and females of series II and III. There were then at least twenty cages each of series I males and females and series II males and females and at least ten cages each of series III males and females. Twenty cages of series I males were allocated to the five tanks using tables of random numbers with the restriction that each tank was to have four cages. Similar random allocation was made of all the other experimental mice, so that each tank contained four series I, four series II and two series III cages of each sex. Allocation was made at weaning time seven weeks before the mice were put into the tanks. A few mice died within the first week after weaning and were replaced by spares of the appropriate series, which had been kept for the purpose. The sexes were segregated throughout. On the day irradiation started the mice were 11 to 13½ weeks old (mean age, 90 days).

It is believed that the allocation of mice between the different experimental groups was entirely unbiased. No mice were excluded from the process of allocation because they were undersized or for any other reason, so that each group consisted of a random sample of CBA mice which had survived five weeks from birth.

3. CHOICE OF DOSE RATE

It was originally proposed to have a maximum dose rate of fast neutrons of 2 rads per day which would have been expected to kill all the mice in about six months, assuming an r.b.e. of 10 (cf. Henshaw,

1944; Henshaw *et al.*, 1947; Lorenz *et al.*, 1947). The other two areas available for fast neutron exposures were to be used for a medium dose rate of about one-tenth and a minimum dose rate of about one-thirtieth of the maximum. If the r.b.e. were 10 the medium dose rate would approximate to the gamma ray exposure of 2·2 r daily of Lorenz *et al.* (1947), which appeared to produce a just detectable excess of deaths over the controls beginning at about the time that half the controls had died (for this analysis of the data of Lorenz *et al.*, 1947, see Mole, 1948, and Sampford, 1952). The minimum dose rate of fast neutrons would not then have been expected to have any detectable effect. If the r.b.e. were really 30 or 40 for long-term effects, as has been suggested (for summary of data see Mitchell, 1952), the minimum dose rate would have been expected to have the same effect as 2·2 r daily of gamma rays, i.e. to be just detectable and the medium dose rate to have a correspondingly more obvious effect.

The proposed dose rates for fast neutrons therefore seemed to be those which would produce the greatest amount of useful information on the reasonable assumption that the gamma ray experiment of Lorenz *et al.* provided representative information on the chronic radio-sensitivity of mice. The maximum dose rate in fact achieved was about 1 rad/day, for reasons discussed elsewhere (Chap. I, §9 (i) (a), p. 14), but the relative dose rates in the three exposure areas were not altered.

4. CONTINUITY OF IRRADIATION

The great advantage of the experimental arrangement was that the mice could be irradiated almost continuously, and it was hoped to have the irradiation of the animals spread as evenly as possible throughout the week. In order to have some control over the dose rate other than altering the running power of the pile, a system of shutters was installed between the pile reflector and the uranium under the animal cages (see Fig. 2, Chap. I, §8, p. 10).

Although the pile was expected to run at a constant power level as far as could be foreseen, planning for a 24-hour exposure every day of the week was impracticable since it was clearly impossible to predict for two years ahead when and for how long the pile would be shut down. In fact during the construction period when the concrete shielding of the pile was being modified to take the animals and the irradiation facilities were being built, other work with the pile necessitated a considerable increase in running power for one or two days a week. By closing the shutters underneath the animal tanks during most of these days, but opening them for short times as required, the daily dose could be kept from rising too high and the weekly dose kept approximately constant. During the rest of the week at the lower pile power it was intended to keep the shutters open for 16 hours a day. Even with the shutters shut at the lower pile power the animals received an appreciable amount of radiation (Table 1) and the number of hours per week entirely free of irradiation was to be determined by the weekly shut-down for servicing of the pile.

Fourteen months after the start of the experiment the period of high-power running of the pile was increased to three days per week. To avoid an increase in the weekly dose from the unavoidable background fast neutrons (Chap. I, §9 (ii), p. 17), it was necessary to remove the animals from the irradiation areas for one whole day a week. The fluctuations in dose from day to day and the number of hours per week entirely free from irradiation therefore increased from this point (Figs. 12 and 13).

5. CONTAMINATING RADIATIONS

In practice, fast neutrons produced by nuclear fission in uranium are accompanied by thermal neutrons and gamma rays. The thermal neutron doses were easily reduced to biologically insignificant levels (Chap. I, §9 (iii), p. 18). There was a limit, however, to the reduction of gamma radiation (Chap. I, §9, p. 13), and for practical purposes it was decided to regard the fast neutrons as pure if less than five per cent. of the biological effect produced could be attributed to contaminating gamma radiation. This criterion involved the use of some assumption about the r.b.e. of neutrons as compared with

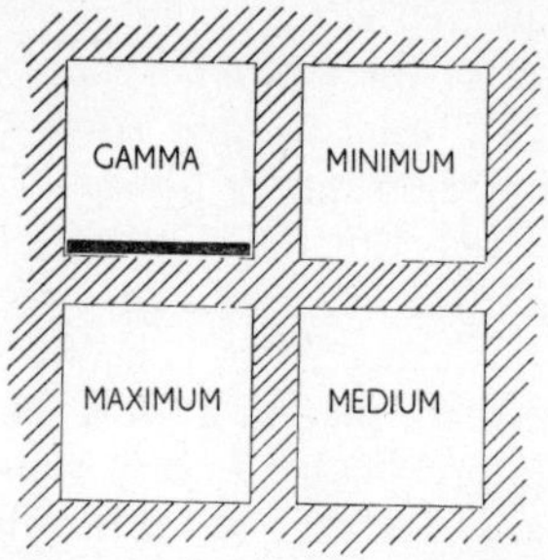

FIG. 1. Schematic plan view of experimental tanks.
▬▬ paraffin wax (Chap. I, §9 (i), p. 17).

	Dose rates in the tanks (Table 19)			
	MAXIMUM	MEDIUM	MINIMUM	GAMMA
Fast neutrons (rads/week)	6·4	0·54	0·19	0·08
Gamma rays (r/week)	1·6	0·84	0·98	0·67

gamma rays. In the tank with the maximum neutron dose rate (MAXIMUM tank Fig. 1) the criterion was met even though the r.b.e. were assumed to be as low as 5. In the MEDIUM tank (Fig. 1) about 13 per cent of any biological effect produced could be attributed to the gamma radiation, assuming an r.b.e. of 10. In the MINIMUM tank (Fig. 1), the gamma contribution was about 35 per cent assuming the same r.b.e. If the r.b.e. were really more than 10, the relative effect of the gamma contamination would have been smaller than the figures given and vice versa. In any case, the actual weekly gamma ray dose rates were less than twice the human maximum permissible level except in the MAXIMUM tank.

6. ANIMAL CARE

The successful outcome of any experiment lasting for the duration of an animal's lifetime depends primarily on the standards of hygiene and animal care employed. Short of an epidemic in the ordinary sense of the word, infective illnesses would increase the uncontrolled variability of the results, as measured by shortening of life span. Nutrition, air temperature, the degree of crowding in the cages and other less tangible factors would also be expected to be important. These general considerations had already led to the conclusion that experimental tunnels were never likely to be satisfactory sources of radiation. An arrangement by which animals lived their whole lives in the place where they were irradiated seemed essential, and was achieved as described later.

Four irradiation areas, 4¼ ft. square, were available, and in each of these it was just possible to accommodate the desired minimum number of 100 mice, housed in 20 aluminium cages, 10 × 8 × 5 in., five mice per cage. Previous experience had shown that with five mice in this size of cage there was no overcrowding, and a cage could be left for seven days without changing the sawdust.

The routine of animal care was to change all the animals of one of the five tanks from soiled cages into clean sterilized cages on a fixed day of each week. One cage was dealt with at a time, and the mice weighed individually at the time of transfer. Mice once caged together were thus left together throughout and the chances of transfer of an infective agent from one cage to another were minimized. The soiled cages were removed from the pile building without their contents being further disturbed. The cages had solid sides to decrease the chances of transfer of infection from one cage to another while in the exposure tanks: the lids were perforated to allow exchange of air.

All the mice were fed on the same batches of a standard cubed ration (Rat Nut 14 per cent, North Eastern Agricultural Co-operative Society Ltd.) filled into a hopper built into the cages. They were given chlorinated water to drink from 8-oz. bottles which were replaced once weekly by fresh, sterilized bottles. There was a daily inspection, including weekends, of food hoppers and bottles, which could be examined without opening the cages. During the first year bottles occasionally leaked away into cages sometimes making them very wet inside, but with serious effects on one occasion only. As defective drinking tubes were eliminated this occurred increasingly rarely.

The four irradiated groups were in adjacent steel tanks sunk in a large mass of concrete, and as might have been expected, the air temperatures inside them were the same. Each tank was covered by a movable shield (Chap. I, §8, p. 10). The four shields were the same size and symmetrically placed. The air in each tank was in free communication with the air of the pile building through spaces of the same size and shape between the top surface of the pile and the under surface of the shields, and since each tank held the same number of mice* it is believed that the air in the tanks had the same relative humidity and the same content of ammonia, acetamide and other volatile materials. The lids of the cages were perforated and the shields cut off most of the light. Thus all the mice were in the same degree of semi-darkness, except for a short period daily when the shutters were opened for inspection of food hoppers and water bottles, and during a longer period once weekly when the change into clean cages was made.

The spaces between the shields, and between the shields and the upper surface of the pile concrete were covered in by wire netting in order to prevent wild mice or rats from getting into the tanks and possibly infecting the experimental mice. In the event no trace of such wild rodents was ever found on the top face of the concrete shield of the pile.

The fifth (CONTROL) tank was constructed exactly like the other four and was built out over the edge of the top face of the pile. The mice in this tank received no measurable dose of radiation. Its sides and bottom were given a double wall and through the air space thus enclosed, air was circulated by an air conditioning unit. The lid of this tank was made so that there was the same air gap all the way round as there was between the shields of the other four tanks and the top surface of the pile, in order to allow the same degree of inter-

* As cages became empty by the death of the mice in them new batches of animals were put into the tanks (see Chap. I, §7, p. 9), so that during the first two years no tank contained less than 60 mice, except, for a few weeks, the MAXIMUM tank.

change of tank air and air in the pile building. Thus the unirradiated mice had the same routine care as, and lived in conditions identical with the irradiated mice except for very small differences in air temperature (Chap. III, §1 (ii), p. 91).

After the experiment had been running for 14 months it became necessary to remove the animals from the tanks for one day a week if their weekly dose was not to be increased (Chap. I, §4, p. 6). A large box was built on part of the unused concrete of the top pile face enclosing a floor area of about 10 ft. square, so as to accommodate all the cages from the four irradiated tanks (Fig. 3). Since the air temperature on the top face of the pile in summer sometimes rose to more than 95°F, some 25°F above the temperature of the air in the tanks set in the concrete of the pile, it was necessary to control the temperature of the box. This was done in a similar manner to the CONTROL tank by giving it a double wall through which air was circulated by a thermostatically controlled air conditioning unit.

7. OBSERVATION OF RADIATION EFFECTS

As already mentioned, shortening of life span seemed the most sensitive index of chronic radiation damage, so that the main experimental record was of the day of death of each mouse. For various reasons this decision imposed limitations on the additional information which could be gained from the same groups of animals. It was recognized that the additional trauma and handling in such procedures as obtaining blood counts, examining the eye for cataract, or palpating the animal for tumours might effect survival and must therefore be avoided. Allowing animals to die implied that post-mortem examinations would be of limited value, and preservation of tissues for histological examination poor. The only additional observation which would not interfere with the main purpose of the experiment was the determination of the weight of each animal once weekly during transfer from a soiled to a clean cage at the time when handling was inevitable. The appearance of visible tumours was recorded at the same time.

For the first ten months of the experiment the cages were inspected for dead mice only when there was olfactory evidence that a mouse was indeed dead. As soon as animals in the MAXIMUM tank began to die the cages were inspected daily for deaths.

When the main experiment had been set up and twenty mouse cages had been placed in each tank, there was just room in each tank for four more cages, each half the size of the standard type. These small cages were of an unusual shape, and very deep for their area. Subsequent experience (Chap. III, §2 (ii), p. 107), suggested that living conditions were not as good as in the standard cage even when the volume of cage space per mouse was greater. The reason is likely to have been the poorer ventilation of the narrow deep cages with consequent increases in temperature, humidity and concentration of volatile materials.

It was decided to utilize the small cages for subsidiary experiments, and initially to test the effect of fast neutrons on fertility and on cataract in the same mice. Preliminary results showed that male sterility was produced in a few weeks by a dose of neutrons which did not produce lens opacities in several months (Neary, Munson and Mole, 1953). Sterilization of male mice therefore seemed a more sensitive index of radiation damage than cataract formation, and intensive observations on cataract were not made. As well as providing data on fertility of male and female mice, the small cages were used for mice which were deliberately killed at various time intervals to provide information on blood counts, on the weights of organs, and on histological changes in tissues where post-mortem changes could be excluded. As soon as space was available, cages of the standard size were used instead of the small cages for these additional observations.

8. GENERAL STRUCTURAL LAY-OUT

The smaller pile (GLEEP) at the Atomic Energy Research Establishment seemed suitable for a chronic irradiation experiment because

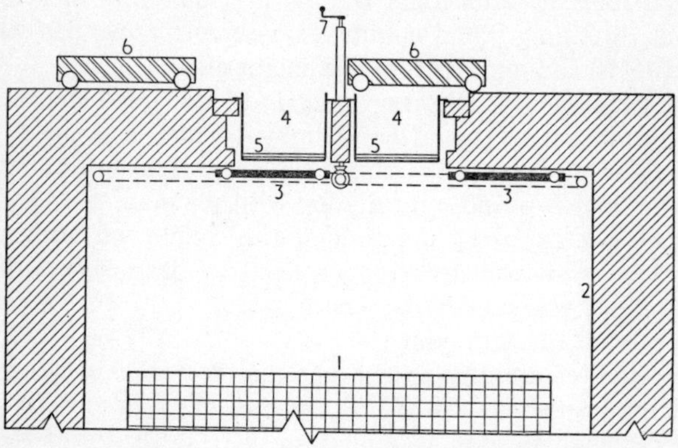

FIG. 2. Schematic drawing of a vertical section through the pile to show the general arrangement of the irradiation tanks.

1. Graphite of pile
2. Concrete shield of pile
3. Shutters
4. Irradiation tanks
5. Uranium and other materials (details in Fig. 4).
6. Movable shields
7. Operating handle for movement of shutter

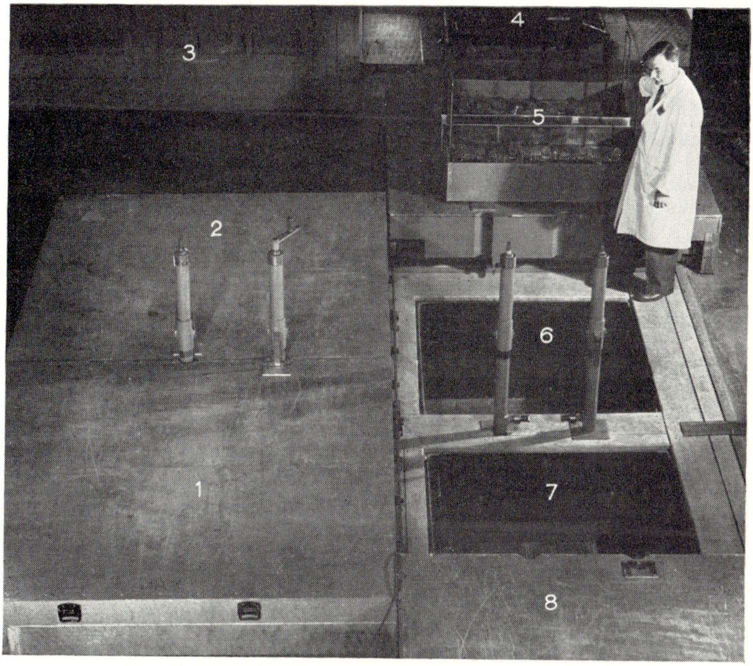

FIG. 3. Photograph of top face of GLEEP, showing the irradiation and control tanks

1. Movable shield over MAXIMUM tank
2. Movable shield over GAMMA tank
3. Control box (temperature-controlled)
4. CONTROL tank
5. Trays containing animal cages from MINIMUM tank resting on movable shield of tank
6. MINIMUM tank
7. MEDIUM tank
8. Movable shield of MEDIUM tank

it was expected normally to run continuously at a constant power level. The top face of the pile was not required for other experimental purposes, and the concrete shield of this face afforded a satisfactory working space. Fig. 2 is a schematic drawing of a vertical section through the top shield of the pile and Fig. 3 a photograph showing the general arrangement. A centrally situated hole, about 12 ft. square, in the shield could be opened up by the removal of concrete plugs, thereby exposing the top surface of the graphite reflector of the pile about 12 ft. below. A preliminary experiment at the then normal operating power of the pile, 300 watts, showed that the thermal neutron flux at the level of the inner or lower surface of the shield was about 10^5 neutrons/cm^2/second, and that the conversion of this thermal flux in a layer of natural uranium led to a fast neutron dose of about 2 rads per 24 hours. The large hole in the shield was divided into four smaller holes about 4½ ft. square separated by means of steel and concrete girders about 1 ft. thick, so that radiations in one hole should not reach the other holes. Different neutron dose levels could then be maintained in three of the holes. The fourth hole was intended to have no neutron radiation and to serve as a control, since it was known that in each hole there would be an unavoidable small background of gamma radiation amounting to about 0·2 r per day. Into each of the four holes, a strong metal tank was fitted, with sides of steel and base of reinforced aluminium to transmit thermal neutrons. The tops of the tanks were flush with the top surface of the concrete shield, while their bases were 10 in. higher than the bottom surface of the concrete shield, the thickness of which was 4 ft.

It was desirable to be able to interrupt the fast neutron irradiation in each tank without shutting the pile down so that the animals could be serviced without hazardous exposure and so that there could be some control over the dose to the animals. The simplest procedure seemed to be to stop the formation of fast neutrons in the uranium of a tank by preventing the thermal neutrons from entering. Therefore movable shutters which could absorb thermal neutrons were provided underneath each tank. The shutters consisted of trays about 1 in. in depth filled with a mixture of equal parts of borax and paraffin wax. They moved on horizontal rails and their tops were almost level with the bottom surface of the concrete shield; each was of area sufficient to cover, with a few inches overlap, the hole into which a tank was fitted. The shutters could be controlled individually from outside the pile shield, and any or all tanks could be completely screened or unscreened from the thermal neutrons. When a shutter was in the closed position, the thermal neutron flux reaching the base of the corresponding tank was negligible.

In order to prevent the fast neutrons from the tanks from causing a radiation hazard in the working area on top of the pile, each tank was provided with a massive shield filled with paraffin wax or sawdust. The individual shields could be moved aside on runners in order to permit access to the animals in the tanks, but shields and shutters were interlocked mechanically so that both shield and shutter of the same tank could not be open simultaneously.

9. THE RADIATIONS IN THE TANKS

The basic physical requirements were:

(1) to provide fast neutron dose levels of approximately two rads per day, one-tenth of this figure, and one-thirtieth of this figure in three tanks respectively;

(2) to ensure uniformity of dose over the area of a tank;

(3) to reduce gamma radiation and slow neutrons to negligible amounts.

The fast neutrons were produced in three tanks by conversion of thermal neutrons by fission in uranium at the bottom of each tank. The two lower dose rates were obtained by reducing the thermal

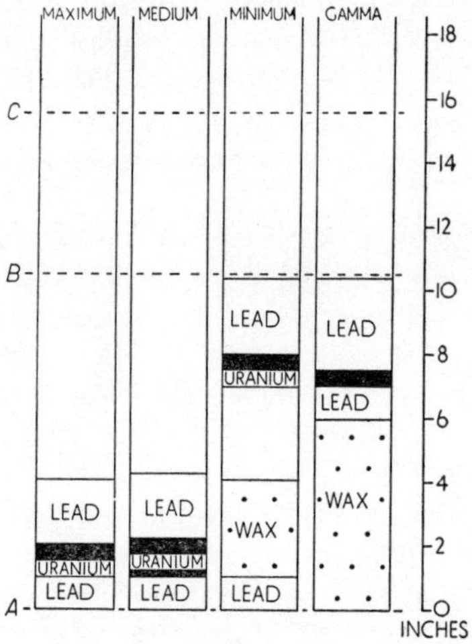

FIG. 4. Schematic vertical section of experimental tanks showing the various layers of lead, uranium, etc. Black shading indicates thermal neutron absorbers of boron carbide above the uranium, and of boron glass below the uranium in the MEDIUM tank

A Level of base of tanks
B Level of bottoms of the animal cages
C Level of lids of cages

fluxes to the desired levels by attenuators below the uranium (see Fig. 4).

In view of the expected biological variability of the mice, it was thought unnecessary to reduce the range of dose variation in a tank to less than about 10 per cent of the mean value.

As regards the contaminating gamma and slow neutron radiations to which the mice would be exposed, it was thought desirable to reduce these to the commonly accepted maximum permissible levels. The reduction of the thermal neutron fluxes to very low levels presented no technical difficulty, but the reduction of gamma radiation, by means of a heavy absorber such as lead, involved also a reduction of the fast neutrons and a degradation of their energy by scattering.

(i) *Fast Neutron Radiation*

The thermal neutron flux available for conversion in the uranium in the tanks at a pile power of 300 watts was of the order of 10^5 neutrons per cm^2 per second, as deduced from the current in a boron trifluoride chamber. The flux was by no means uniform over the area of the tanks, tending to be lower at points further from the central region of the pile; the fall-off was more pronounced in directions perpendicular to the channel axis of the pile than in longitudinal directions. In addition, there were more rapid and erratic variations from point to point, some of which could be attributed to absorption in the aluminium girders reinforcing the sheet aluminium base of a tank. The flux near the edges of the tanks tended to be low probably because of partial screening by the surrounding concrete, which had to extend below the tanks in order to permit of a satisfactory shutter arrangement. In the MAXIMUM tank it appeared easiest to attempt to attain uniformity of fast neutron dose rate by adjustment of the distribution of uranium over the area of the tank, while in the MEDIUM and MINIMUM tanks, where the thermal flux had to be considerably attenuated, it seemed easiest to adjust the variation of the thermal flux using a practically continuous layer of uranium.

The uranium was in the form of slabs 13 in. long, and 3¼ in. wide. The thickness of the slabs, 2/5 in., was chosen to give a reasonably large utilization of the thermal neutrons while not seriously absorbing and degrading by inelastic scattering fast neutrons produced in the slab. The slabs could be arranged edge to edge in a tank to give a continuous layer over the whole area, but some alteration in the distribution was made in each tank in order to attain the desired uniformity of fast neutron dose. Each uranium slab was coated with graphite to a thickness of about three-thousandths of an inch by painting on a suspension of colloidal graphite; this layer served to prevent the direct emission of the fission product recoils. The slabs were wrapped in thin aluminium sheet and the joints sealed by 'Sellotape'.

(a) MAXIMUM *Tank*

The fast neutron dose rate at standard power (300 W) with uranium covering the floor of the MAXIMUM tank was about 80 millirads per hour, but varied by 20 per cent or so over the area. Even with a uniform thermal flux, the fast neutron dose rate at the edges of a uniform area of uranium would be expected to be low relative to the centre value. In order to compensate at the edges, a double layer of uranium blocks was used round the edges of the tank and the blocks over the inner part of the area were spaced apart. This general arrangement was successively modified until a satisfactory fast neutron dose distribution was obtained. Details of the intermediate stages need not be given, but it may be mentioned that some narrow strips of cadmium were stuck on the base of the tank in between the reinforcing girders to compensate for the 'shadows' made by the latter. The average fast neutron dose rate over the area with the shutter open was now 62 millirads/hour and the extreme variations were 12 per cent up or down.

When precise measurements had been made in all tanks it was found that background fast neutrons from the pile itself were producing a dose rate of about 1·5 millirads/hour in all tanks. For reasons explained below, this background was unacceptable and various measures were taken to reduce it. For the MAXIMUM tank, it was essential not to lose too many thermal neutrons in the process. In the event, two layers of 7¼-in.-thick graphite blocks were added to the top surface of the graphite reflector, thereby reducing the fast neutron background to about one-fifth the previous value. However, the thermal flux was now considerably reduced, leading to a mean fast neutron dose rate in the tank with its shutter open of about 42 millirads/hour. Minor disturbances of the uniformity had also occurred and these were rectified by alterations to the uranium distribution and to the cadmium strips on the base of the tank.

The effective floor levels in the GAMMA and MINIMUM tanks had been raised about 6 in. by the addition of a layer of paraffin wax (see below), and it was felt that the effective depth of all the tanks should be the same so as to have comparable conditions of ventilation and environment generally. This requirement was satisfied in the MAXIMUM and MEDIUM tanks by providing an aluminium platform 6 in. high resting on top of the upper layers of lead, etc. The depth of the effective floor of all tanks was thus 2 ft. 4 in. below the tops of the tanks.

The distribution of fast neutron dose rate was remeasured at this new level and found to be satisfactory. The mean value was 36·4 millirads/hour (Table 1) and was uniform within about ± 10 per cent.

(b) MEDIUM *Tank*

The dose rate in the MEDIUM tank was intended to be one-tenth that in the MAXIMUM tank. The necessary reduction of the slow neutron flux at the uranium to a value about one-tenth of that in the MAXIMUM tank was effected by glass of high boron content. The density (2·36 g/cm^3) and composition (17 per cent by weight B_2O_3) of the glass were constant; square pieces of $5\frac{3}{4}$ in. side were used, and the thickness was sufficiently uniform over this area. The required thickness of the glass was around 1/5 in., but there was a considerable range of thicknesses so that the slow neutron flux over any given small area of the tank could be adjusted precisely to any required value. In a few cases when the supply of glass of a particular thickness was exhausted, a slightly thinner piece was used and a small fraction of its area made opaque to thermal neutrons by sticking on a piece of cadmium foil.

Thermal neutron fluxes were determined by measuring the current produced in a boron trifluoride chamber. The chamber centre was about 4 cm above the surface of the glass whereas the flux it was desired to measure was the flux at the surface of the glass on which the uranium slabs would lie. It was therefore thought desirable to allow the chamber to respond only to thermal neutrons coming through the glass in its immediate vicinity. A cadmium hood was placed round the chamber, arbitrarily restricting the area that could be 'seen' to $5\frac{3}{4}$ in. square, i.e. one piece of glass. After an initial survey of the unattenuated thermal neutron distribution over the floor of the tank, an arrangement of glass was calculated to give an approximately uniform attenuated thermal neutron distribution, except for the outermost band of $5\frac{3}{4}$ in. in which fluxes estimated at some 50 per cent. greater were required. After the actual distribution had been checked and the glass thickness modified where necessary, the uranium and lead were added (over a 'cushion' of sheet rubber 3/16 in. thick) and the fast neutron dose rate distribution measured. In the light of the result, modifications to the arrangement of glass were made, and after the procedure had been repeated a few times, a satisfactorily uniform distribution of fast neutron dose rate was achieved, the mean value being around 7 millirads/hour.

When the reduction of the background of fast neutrons from the pile came to be considered (see below), it was found not worth while to replace the boron glass attenuator by paraffin wax. Just as in the MAXIMUM tank, an aluminium platform 6 in. high was added on top of the layers of lead, etc. The fast neutron dose rate was now quite different because

(1) the thermal neutron flux had been halved by the two extra layers of graphite on the pile

(2) the fast neutron background from the pile was reduced to about one-fifth, and

(3) the distance from the uranium had been increased by the inclusion of the platform.

The distribution was uniform within about ± 10 per cent, with a mean of 3·0 millirads/hour, (Table 1).

(c) MINIMUM *Tank*

The development of the MINIMUM tank proceeded similarly to that of the MEDIUM tank. The thermal neutron flux reaching the uranium was required to be about one-thirtieth of that in the MAXIMUM tank, and so, at first, glass of about 3/10 in. in thickness was used as an attenuator. The fast neutron dose rate, using an approximately continuous layer of uranium, was about 3·3 millirads/hour instead of the expected value of about 1·6 millirads/hour. When the amount of uranium was halved, the dose rate fell to about 2·3 millirads/hour. These results were explicable when further measurements showed that there was a background of fast neutrons from the pile in all tanks equal to about 1·5 millirads/hour (see below). Ultimately, the boron glass attenuator was replaced by a tray 6 in. deep containing a 3-in. layer of paraffin wax. The layer of uranium was approximately continuous, with minor variations to ensure sufficient uniformity of fast neutron dose rate. The mean value of the dose rate was 0·9 millirads/hour (Table 1) and the variations were mostly within ± 10 per cent.

(d) GAMMA *Tank*

The purpose of the GAMMA tank was to expose mice to the same level of gamma radiation as was present as a contaminant in the three 'neutron' tanks. The GAMMA tank differed from the other three tanks principally in that it contained no uranium as no fast neutrons were required. The original arrangement for this tank was a 1-in. layer of lead at the bottom, a boron carbide layer to stop thermal neutrons, followed by a 2-in. layer of lead. The tank was provided with a thermal neutron shutter underneath. Before introduction of the modifications needed to reduce the fast neutron background from the pile (see below), a satisfactory match had been achieved between the gamma radiation levels in the GAMMA, the MINIMUM and the MEDIUM tanks, viz about 5 mr/hour with shutters open and 2·2 mr/hour with shutters closed. The gamma level in the MAXIMUM tank was roughly twice as high, but in this tank the gamma radiation was negligible in comparison with the fast neutron radiation (see Table 1).

After the experimental arrangement had been reorganized so as to reduce the pile fast neutron background, it was decided to keep the GAMMA tank shutter always closed in order to take advantage of the slight extra reduction of fast neutron background thereby, even though this entailed a slightly lower gamma dose level in the GAMMA tank than in the other tanks.

It was found that when the shutter of the MAXIMUM tank was open, too many fast neutrons were transmitted from this tank through the concrete beam into the adjoining GAMMA tank. These neutrons were reduced to a satisfactory level by a vertical wall of paraffin wax 10 in. high and 3 in. thick along the side of the tank facing the MAXIMUM tank (Fig. 1).

(ii) *Background Fast Neutron Radiation*

The existence of a background dose in all the tanks due to fast neutron radiation from the pile and equal to about one-fortieth of the total neutron dose in the MAXIMUM tank, was established when the first experimental arrangement was completed and precise measurements were made. Such a background was objectionable because the GAMMA tank would not be free from fast neutron radiation, and further, it was thought that the mean energy of these neutrons might well be different from the 'proper' fast neutrons produced in the three 'neutron' tanks. A much more serious objection was that at this time other work with the pile required a departure from the originally planned programme of continuous running at a constant power of around 300 watts. The programme was now to increase the power on two days per week to 2 kilowatts. The background fast neutrons would be little reduced by the closing of the thermal neutron shutters, and consequently the period of high power running would lead to a substantial and roughly equal contribution to the dose rate in all four tanks; the total dose rates would therefore not be in the desired ratios.

Experiments with various thicknesses of water barriers below and at the sides of an ionization chamber suggested that most of the background neutrons were coming directly from the pile, and that scattering from the concrete shields was not important. There were three unplugged vertical holes through the reflector and directly below the experimental tanks; their diameters were about $3\frac{1}{2}$ in. It was shown that when these holes were covered with water tanks, the background was only slightly reduced and it was therefore concluded that the smaller and more remote holes for the control and shut-off rods were not responsible for any large part of the background. It seemed likely that the background neutrons were transmitted through the reflector generally, and did not escape from particular holes in the pile.

Attempts were then made to shield the animals from the background neutrons by putting barriers of slowing-down material in the bottoms of the tanks. A layer of 5½ in. of paraffin wax in the GAMMA tank reduced the background to about one-eighth. In the MINIMUM tank only 3 in. of paraffin wax could be used because of the loss of thermal neutrons. In the MEDIUM and MAXIMUM tanks the use of paraffin wax as a slowing down medium was impracticable because of the loss of thermal neutrons by reflection and capture, while the use of graphite appeared to take up too much space. It was therefore decided to lay extra graphite on top of the pile itself. One layer of graphite 7¼ in. thick was placed over the easily accessible part of the area which was about two-thirds the total, and the residual background immediately over this layer was investigated. It was shown that additional side walls and roof of 7¼ in. graphite blocks around the ionization chamber did not further reduce the background, but an additional floor did so by a factor of about two. A second layer of 7¼ in. of graphite was therefore added on top of the first. The total effect of the two layers of graphite was to reduce the background fast neutrons to about one-fifth, but to reduce the thermal flux reaching the tanks to about one-half. This arrangement was accepted as satisfactory.

It should be emphasized that the figures quoted for the attenuating effect of the various barriers on the fast neutrons are approximate. The measurements were made in a hurry because the mice were now ready and there was a considerable background of gamma rays and thermal neutrons, which could not be adequately removed in the rough experimental 'lash-ups'. In the measurement of the final values of the dose rates of the background neutrons in the tanks, the backgrounds of gamma rays and thermal neutrons were small and did not seriously affect the measurements.

(iii) *Thermal Neutrons*

In order to stop those thermal neutrons not absorbed in the uranium, there was a layer of boron carbide immediately above the layer of uranium. Boron was chosen in preference to cadmium because of the much more easily absorbed gamma ray of 0·478 MeV produced at slow neutron capture and because, unlike cadmium, boron also absorbs epithermal neutrons. The absorber had to be in the form of a robust sheet to withstand frequent handling and removal from a tank during the frequent rearrangements of the attenuator and uranium layer, and to be free from spilling of the boron carbide. It was therefore constructed by rivetting together two sheets of 10-gauge aluminium held 5 mm apart by aluminium spacing pieces round the edges and at a few places over the area. The boron carbide was then poured into the sandwich through a small hole which was later sealed. In this way a mean thickness corresponding to 0·75 g/cm^2 of boron carbide was obtained, but even with this comparatively large thickness a few small 'holes' due to bad packing were apparent when the transmission of thermal neutrons was examined. Therefore the upper surface of the boron carbide absorber was covered with a thin sheet of cadmium to ensure the removal of the few neutrons passing through the holes in the boron carbide. The small additional production of hard gamma rays was unimportant. Details are given in Table 1 below of the final thermal neutron fluxes reaching the mice in the individual tanks. These values include the thermal neutrons produced by the slowing down of some of the fast neutrons. The highest flux was in the MAXIMUM tank and it was estimated to be biologically equivalent to about one-tenth of the maximum permissible dose of gamma rays and was therefore negligible.

(iv) *Gamma Radiation*

The unwanted gamma radiation in a tank arose from six different sources:

1. the pile itself, irradiating the bases of all four tanks practically uniformly.
2. capture of slow neutrons in the boron glass or paraffin wax attenuator used (in the MEDIUM and MINIMUM tanks).
3. the uranium (a) due to its natural radioactivity, (b) during absorption of slow neutrons in fission and capture processes, (c) due to the fission products formed in (b).
4. capture in the boron carbide stopper of slow neutrons not absorbed in the uranium.
5. capture of slow neutrons in the steel walls of a tank and in the surrounding concrete, especially with the shutter open. This radiation was reduced by filling the narrow gap between the steel tanks and the concrete with lead. The gap was not everywhere the same, but thicknesses of one-half to one inch of lead were inserted.
6. inelastic scattering of fast neutrons in the tank.

Since most of the gamma ray emission from fission products in the uranium is associated with those products with half-lives not much greater than a few seconds, the emission of this radiation may, for the present purposes, be regarded as instantaneous just as that due to fission and capture. Thus the gamma radiation arising in the uranium of a given tank has a constant component (natural radioactivity) and a component dependent on the opening of the thermal neutron shutter below the tank, and which is proportional to the fission rate in the tank and therefore to the fast neutron dose rate in the tank. Similarly, the intensity of the gamma rays due to slow neutron capture in the boron carbide stopper is proportional to the slow neutron flux transmitted through the uranium, which in turn is proportional to the fast neutron dose rate in the tank, and is negligible when the shutter is closed.

It is apparent therefore that the production of gamma radiation is different in the different tanks, the differences being greater when the shutters are open. It was thought desirable to reduce the gamma radiation reaching the animals in all four tanks to comparable amounts and if possible to 'tolerance' level. As mentioned already, the thickness of lead which may be used for such shielding is limited owing to the degradation of neutron energy which also occurs in the lead, and by practical considerations of weight. The desirability of having the same distribution of neutron energies in all three 'neutron' tanks entails having the same thickness of lead absorber on top of the uranium in these tanks. Further the desirability of reducing the degradation of neutron energy to the minimum, and the fact that some gamma radiation comes from places below the uranium and boron carbide neutron stopper, implies that some of the total available lead should be used underneath the uranium. It was nevertheless clear that a substantial proportion of the total lead to be used would have to be on top of the uranium and boron carbide because of the large differences in gamma radiation production in these components in the three 'neutron' tanks. Ideally, such radiation should be reduced to such small levels as to be negligible compared to the other sources of gamma radiation which were more or less the same for all tanks, i.e. pile radiation and capture radiation in concrete, steel, etc. It was clear that the gamma radiation from the uranium (and much less importantly from the boron carbide) would follow on the average much more oblique paths through the overlying lead absorber than would that from the pile, etc., and so would suffer a considerably greater relative reduction. Consequently, it was practicable to reduce the gamma radiation from the uranium to very low levels and thus ensure that the total gamma radiation doses in the different tanks were similar.

The allocation of lead could only be decided rather roughly because of the difficulty of measuring accurately the levels of gamma radiation and fast neutrons in the presence of a high flux of slow neutrons. After trial and error, it was concluded that a layer of one inch of lead beneath the uranium and two inches on top gave a satisfactory arrangement.

It was originally intended to use boron in the form of boron plate glass for the slow neutron attenuators in both the MEDIUM and the MINIMUM tanks. There would have been a very small transmission of the capture gamma radiation from boron through the overlying uranium and two inches of lead, and so it was thought unnecessary to place the attenuator below the lowest one-inch layer of lead.

In the final arrangement the gamma ray dose rates in the MEDIUM and MINIMUM tanks were not quite the same, because different thermal neutron attenuators were used. At a late stage in the work, it was found necessary to replace the boron glass attenuator in the MINIMUM tank by a 3-in. layer of paraffin wax in order to reduce the background fast neutrons from the pile (Chap. 1, §9 (ii), p. 17). The gamma radiation due to capture of slow neutrons in paraffin is much less readily absorbed in lead than the capture radiation from boron and so the level of gamma rays in the MINIMUM tank became higher. It would therefore have been preferable to place the paraffin below the lowest layer of lead, but owing to the urgency of completing the arrangement to receive the young mice, this modification was not made. In consequence, the gamma radiation level to which animals in the MINIMUM tank were exposed, though negligible considered absolutely ($\sim 0{\cdot}1$ r/day), was nevertheless slightly higher than in the MEDIUM tank (Table 1). The shutter below the GAMMA tank was always kept closed and so the capture gamma radiation from the paraffin in this tank was negligible. Capture gamma radiation from the shutters was predominantly due to boron and not to the hydrogen of the wax in the shutters.

The gamma radiation dose rate in the MAXIMUM tank was about twice that in the other tanks but this excess was unimportant in comparison with the high neutron dose rate in this tank.

10. DOSE LEVELS IN THE TANKS

Dose measurements were normally made with the chamber centres at a height of 4 cm above the effective floor of a tank. The rate of fall off of fast neutron dose rate with height was about $2\frac{1}{2}$ per cent per centimetre. The position of the ionization chambers during dose measurements was thus a close approximation to the position of the mice during irradiation, since the latter were contained in boxes with about $1\frac{1}{4}$ cm of bedding in the bottom, and the boxes rested in an aluminium tray. A separate experiment was made with all the animals in the tank but with one mouse box containing the ionization chambers and some dummy mice. The fast neutron dose rate under these conditions was about 1½ per cent less than the corresponding 'in air' dose rate, while the gamma ray dose rate was about 2 per cent less. It has not been thought worth while to correct the 'in air' measurements by these small amounts, which are barely significant.

The radiation levels in the tanks at a standard pile power of 300 watts are given in Table 1. The levels of fast neutron dose rates above the movable tank shield when the shutter was open were about 8 per cent of the values in the tank for the GAMMA, MINIMUM and MEDIUM tanks, and about 3 per cent for the MAXIMUM tank.

TABLE 1

Radiation levels at 300 *watts*

Tank: Designation	Tank: Shutter position	Shutter under MAXIMUM tank	Fast neutrons (millirads per hour)	Gamma rays (milliroentgens per hour)	Thermal (neutrons (n/cm²/sec)
MAXIMUM	Open		36·4±0·7	6·95±0·7	1480±30
	Closed		0·77±0·08	1·56±0·04	40±0·8
MEDIUM	Open	Open	3·02±0·10	2·78±0·07	444±9
		Closed	2·71±0·10	2·48±0·07	377±7
	Closed	Open	0·57±0·08	1·50±0·04	90±2
		Closed	0·30±0·08	1·25±0·04	23±0·4
MINIMUM	Open		0·92±0·08	3·50±0·04	262±5
	Closed		0·20±0·08	1·55±0·04	14±0·2
GAMMA	Closed	Open	0·31±0·08	1·55±0·04	12±0·2
		Closed	0·11±0·08	1·40±0·04	

The errors quoted are the random errors only; they do not include the systematic errors (Chap. II, §12, p. 52) or the spatial variation over the tank.

The position of the shutter below the MAXIMUM tank affected the dose rate in the adjoining MEDIUM and GAMMA tanks for reasons given in the text (Chap I) §9 (i, d), p. 17).

The fast neutron dose rate in the MAXIMUM tank with the shutter closed is higher than the corresponding figure in the MEDIUM tank owing to some small leakage of thermal neutrons through or round the shutter.

Since the pile could not in practice be run continuously at a fixed power, it was arranged that the pile operators would record full details of the actual pile power together with details of the times when the individual shutters of the tanks were opened or closed. As a further check on these records, the actual thermal fluxes between the shutter and the base of each of the four tanks were measured continuously by small boron trifluoride chambers, the outputs of which were passed through amplifiers to a multi-pen recorder.

11. THE ENERGY OF THE NEUTRONS

The biological effects of the neutrons in this experiment were partly determined by their energies. In the first place, there is in general an intrinsic dependence on energy of a given biological effect related to the specific ionization of the radiation; and in the second place, there is a dependence for purely physical reasons which determine the distribution of radiation throughout the body of the animal.

The neutrons from the fission of Uranium 235 have a continuous distribution of energies extending to higher than 10 MeV (*Nucleonics*, 1951). The mean of this distribution is at 2·0 MeV and the median at 1·6 MeV. It was to be expected that the neutrons in this experiment would suffer appreciable degradation of energy in inelastic scattering in the uranium and lead, and by reflection from the shields covering the tanks. The intrinsic biological efficiency of neutrons would not be expected to change much for energies below 2 MeV (Gray, 1946; and Mitchell, 1947). The effect on distribution of radiation in a small animal like a mouse due to a reduction of the mean energy below 2 MeV would not be very marked (see below). Nevertheless, it was desirable to have some approximate information as to how far the neutron radiation to which our mice were exposed differed from the unmodified fission spectrum. An additional consideration is that such information leads to more exact dose estimates (see Chap. II).

One method for estimating the mean neutron energy was suggested by Dr. J. H. Tait of the Theoretical Physics Division, A.E.R.E. The principle is to expose a paraffin sphere to the fast neutrons and to determine the thermal neutron flux inside the sphere at various radial distances. The form of the radial variation of thermal flux depends in a fairly sensitive manner on the energy of the incident fast neutrons. Detailed calculations were carried out (Mandl, 1952) for neutron energies of 0·1, 0·3, 1·0, 2·0 and 3·0 MeV, and a paraffin sphere of 26 cm diameter. For the experimental determinations a paraffin sphere of this diameter divided into two hemispherical pieces was used. Thin manganese foils each 1 cm square were laid flat in the diametral plane between the hemispheres with their centres along a single diameter at positions about 2 cm apart. The beta ray activity of a manganese foil after exposure of the sphere to the fast neutrons was a measure of the thermal flux in the sphere at the position occupied by the foil. Relative activities were determined in a standard set-up with a G-M.4 counter, and suitable corrections were made for radioactive decay and for variations in sensitivity of the foils. It was expected that the fast neutron radiation in the experimental tanks would be approximately isotropic, at least, in the solid angle of 2π below the horizontal plane, and so the diameter along which the foils were spaced was horizontal. The sphere, enclosed in cadmium, was exposed in the MAXIMUM tank with the shutter open and the shield closed and the results indicated an equivalent fast neutron energy of about 0·6 MeV with estimated limits of uncertainty of $\pm$0·15 MeV.

As a check on the method, the sphere was exposed to fast neutrons of known single energy. Dr. M. Poole made available his apparatus giving neutrons of energy 2·9 MeV produced by the $D(d,n)^3He$ reaction, and Dr. D. Allen provided neutrons of 0·6 MeV produced by the $^7Li(p,n)^7Be$ reaction. In both cases, the sphere was exposed to an approximately unidirectional beam, and so to simulate an isotropic irradiation, the sphere was turned into various positions for appropriate intervals during the exposure. The results of these experiments confirmed the theoretical calculations quite closely (Mandl, 1952).

A more detailed investigation of the neutron energies was carried out in collaboration with Mr. R. Batchelor (Batchelor, 1952). The principle of the method is to make use of the reaction $^3He(n,p)^3H$ which is exothermic by 0·77 MeV. The energy of the incident neutron is simply related to the energy of the disintegration proton which is not less than 0·58 MeV (for a thermal neutron). Moreover, the dependence of the cross section for the reaction on neutron energy is fairly well known. Thus if a chamber containing ^3He and a heavy gas such as xenon (to provide stopping power) is exposed to neutrons, the energy spectrum of the latter may be deduced from a measurement of the size distribution of the ionization pulses produced by the disintegration protons. Observations of this kind were made for the MAXIMUM tank both with the shutter opened and closed. Preliminary results, (Batchelor, 1952) indicated a very marked modification of the primary fission spectrum, and a mean neutron energy in reasonable agreement with the estimate of 0·6 MeV by the first method.

In view of the fact that the above methods would only yield rough estimates of neutron energy it seemed worthwhile to expose some Ilford C2 nuclear plates to obtain the proton recoil spectrum, despite the quantitative uncertainty inherent in this method for energies below 0·5 MeV.

In order to secure reasonably good geometry the plates were

exposed in a vertical plane 6 ft. 6 in. above the centre of the uranium layer of the MAXIMUM tank, although it was realized that, in this position, the energy spectrum of the neutrons was probably somewhat different from that of neutrons near the floor of the tank. The processed plates were examined in a microscope with a ×95 objective (N.A. 1·3) and ×10 Kellner eyepieces fitted with eyepiece graticules. All tracks within 10° of the vertical during exposure were recorded. In order to interpret the energy distribution curve for the recoil protons in terms of the neutron spectrum, a number of correction factors had to be applied. These arose from:

(1) the considerable solid angle subtended by the source at the plate, the mean angle of the incident neutrons being 17° from the vertical,

(2) the angular deviation from the vertical of the accepted recoil protons (maximum 10°),

(3) the fact that some tracks were 'lost' owing to the finite emulsion thickness,

(4) the limitations of depth estimation which resulted in some tracks of short length being accepted as within the required limits of ±10° dip, whereas, in fact, they were outside these limits, and

(5) the change of (n, p) scattering cross section with neutron energy.

The results of the analysis of the first four hundred tracks are shown in Fig. 5. This number is too small to establish the shape of

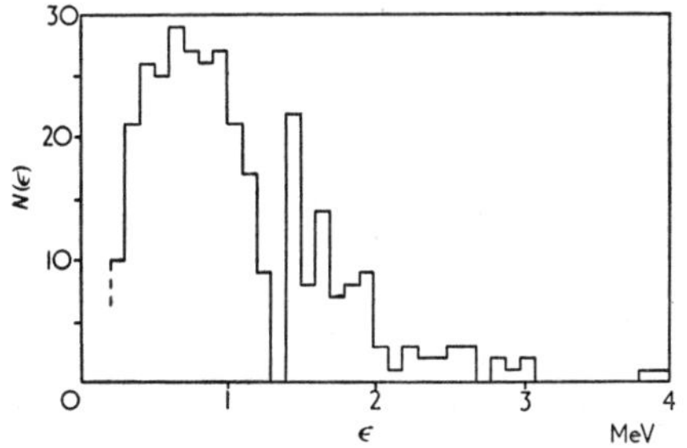

FIG. 5. Neutron energy distribution as given by the lengths of 400 proton recoil tracks in C2 plates.

ϵ = neutron energy (MeV)

$N(\epsilon)$ = number of neutrons in each 0·1 MeV interval

the distribution but at energies above 0·5 MeV, it does seem to conform to the modified fission spectrum, represented by $N(\epsilon) = (8/\pi e)^{\frac{1}{2}} e^{-2\epsilon} \sinh(4\epsilon)^{\frac{1}{2}}$ where ϵ is the neutron energy (Chap. II, §7 (i), p. 38). The proportion of neutrons with energies less than 0·5 MeV appears to be very much smaller than that given by measurement with the ^{3}He chamber and slightly smaller than that for the modified fission spectrum. The mean energy of the neutrons was found to be $1{\cdot}08 \pm 0{\cdot}06$ MeV which is close to the value of 1·0 MeV found from observations with the ^{3}He chamber under similar irradiation conditions, i.e. shutter and shield both open. Both values however, must be regarded as overestimates since neutrons of energy less than 0·2 MeV were excluded by the discriminator bias used with the ^{3}He counter and some of the short proton recoil tracks will have been missed in the scanning of the nuclear plates. Since the measurements with the ^{3}He chamber indicated that the mean energy of the neutrons was reduced by 0·2 MeV on closing the shield, one may conclude that the results of the three methods taken together, give 0·7 MeV for the mean energy of the neutrons reaching the mice under normal irradiation conditions.

12. DOSE DISTRIBUTION IN THE MOUSE

It is important to have some estimate of the variation of fast neutron dose throughout the body of a mouse. The measured doses were the 'in air' doses at the position in the cages occupied by the mice. The actual dose to the under surface of the mice would be increased by backscatter, while the dose to individual organs would depend on the degree of attenuation of the radiation, a factor of possible importance in the assessment of relative biological efficiencies. It was impossible to make experimental measurements of neutron dose distributions with small chambers at the comparatively low dose rates used. A sufficiently good estimate for the interpretation of the biological results was obtained by very approximate considerations.

A mouse of 30 g weight is roughly a cylinder of about $2\frac{1}{2}$ cm diameter and 6 cm length. The mean free path of neutrons of 0·7 MeV, which was the mean energy of the neutrons to which the mice were exposed (this page, above), is 2·2 cm in tissue. In relation to this mean free path, the mouse is therefore neither very small nor very large. Upper and lower limits for the attenuation of dose may be obtained from the data of Tait (1950) for tissue irradiated by narrow and broad beams of fast neutrons, though these refer to normal incidence. The actual irradiation conditions of the mice corresponded more nearly to isotropic incidence but in view of the approximate cylindrical shape of the mouse, there was normal incidence in planes perpendicular to the long axis. From the curves given by Tait (1950), the dose at $1\frac{1}{4}$ cm deep (corresponding to the mid-line of the mouse) as a percentage of the surface dose is 56 per cent for a narrow beam and 82 per cent for a wide beam. An approximate calculation for a sphere of 2·5 cm diameter taking account of the first order scattered radiation only gives a depth dose of 70 per cent at $1\frac{1}{4}$ cm, which agrees with the average of the narrow and wide beam figures. The dose at 2·5 cm deep (corresponding to the full diameter of the mouse) is 32 per cent for the narrow beam and 64 per cent for the wide beam; the average of these figures, 48 per cent agrees with the estimate for a sphere, namely 52 per cent.

It thus seems possible that there was a two-fold variation of neutron dose from the lower to the upper surfaces of the mouse, while the mean dose was about 70 per cent of the dose to the under surface. The ionization chambers measured the air dose with very little attenuation (which is allowed for) or backscatter. According to Tait's data (1950), the percentage surface backscatter is about 16 per cent for a wide beam of 0·7 MeV neutrons. The actual backscatter for a mouse may be about half this figure, i.e. 8 per cent, so the mean dose was about $0{\cdot}7 \times 1{\cdot}08 \times 100 = 75$ per cent of the quoted 'in air' doses.

The distribution of gamma ray dose in the mice would on the other hand be approximately uniform and would correspond to the quoted 'in air' doses.

REFERENCES

BATCHELOR, R., A.E.R.E. Harwell Memorandum, No. N/M 56, 1952.

Biochemical Research Foundation, *Neutron Effects on Animals*, 1947, (ed. ELLICE MCDONALD), Baltimore.

ELY, J. O., ROSS, M. H., METCALFE, R. G., INDA, F. A., BARNETT, T. B., and CASARETT, G. W. in *Biological Effects of External Radiation*, 1954 (ed. H. A. BLAIR), N.N.E.S. VI–2, London.

EVANS, T. C., *Radiology*, 1948, **50**, 811.

EVANS, T. C., *Nucleonics*, 1949, **4**, 2.

GRAY, L. H., *Brit. Med. Bull.*, 1946, **4**, 11.

HENSHAW, P. S., *J. Nat. Cancer Institute*, 1944, **4**, 513.

HENSHAW, P. S., RILEY, E. F., and STAPLETON, G. E., *Radiology*, 1947, **49**, 349.

HENSHAW, P. S., SNIDER, R. S., RILEY, E. F., STAPLETON, G. E., and ZIRKLE, R. E., MDDC 1253, 1946.

LORENZ, E., HESTON, W. E., ESCHENBRENNER, A. B., and DERINGER, M. K., *Radiology*, 1947, **49**, 274.

MANDL, M. E., A.E.R.E. Harwell Report, no. T/R 1008, 1952.

MITCHELL, J. S., *Brit. J. Radiol.*, 1947, **20**, 177.

MITCHELL, J. S., in *Biological Hazards of Atomic Energy*, 1952 (ed. A. HADDOW), Oxford.

MOLE, R. H., Medical Research Council Committee paper NP/P/TD/70, 1948.

NEARY, G. J., MUNSON, R. J., and MOLE, R. H., *Nature*, 1953, **171**, 256.

Nucleonics, 1952, **8**, 78.

SAMPFORD, M. R., *Biometrics*, 1952, **8**, 13 and 307.

TAIT, J. H., *Brit. J. Radiol.*, 1950, **23**, 282.

CHAPTER II

DOSIMETRY

1. INTRODUCTION

ONE of the quantities of fundamental importance in the study of the biological effects of ionizing radiations is the amount of energy absorbed in unit mass of tissue during its exposure. The measurement of this quantity directly, e.g. by calorimetric methods, is normally impracticable and early workers in this field devoted much effort to the practical problem of finding a satisfactory method of estimating radiation doses. This led to the formulation of the definition of the roentgen as a unit of X ray dose, a definition which was later modified to include quantum radiation of higher energy such as gamma rays from radioactive substances. For radiation of a given wavelength the energy absorbed in a small mass of irradiated tissue is proportional to the dose in roentgens.

For the corpuscular radiations such as alpha rays, beta rays and neutrons the rep (roentgen equivalent physical) has been commonly employed as a unit of radiation dose, but in accordance with recent recommendations (*Recommendations of the International Commission on Radiological Units*, 1953) we have expressed our fast neutron doses in rads. In our usage one rad corresponds to an energy absorption of 100 ergs in one gramme of tissue of the composition specified for a 'Standard Man' by the International Commission on Radiological Protection (1955). Gamma ray doses have been given in roentgens.

The energy absorbed in a small mass of a medium exposed to ionizing radiation is independent (within narrow limits) of its physical state. It is therefore possible to deduce the energy absorption in one gramme of tissue from a measurement of the number of ions produced in a known mass of 'tissue-like' gas, if the average energy required to form a pair of ions in this gas is known. This is the basis of our method of estimating fast neutron dose. The separate problem of the distribution of fast neutron dose within a large mass of irradiated tissue has not been considered here.

In practice, the determination of fast neutron dose is usually complicated by the presence of gamma rays. This situation can be met by measuring the ionization current in two chambers of different atomic composition, provided their relative sensitivities to the two types of radiation are known. In using this method, Bretscher and French (1944) employed two geometrically identical chambers, one lined with ordinary paraffin wax and filled with ethylene and the other lined with 'heavy' paraffin wax and filled with deutero-ethylene (C_2D_4). These chambers were thus approximately homogeneous, the walls of each having a composition closely matching that of the gas. Dainty (1950) used strictly homogeneous chambers, one of polythene–ethylene and the other of polystyrene–acetylene. An alternative method recently described by Hurst (1954) involves the use of a homogeneous proportional counter filled with ethylene. The amplifier is biassed to eliminate the relatively small pulses from gamma rays and only the pulses from the more energetic neutron recoils contribute to the measured ionization current.

In our work appreciable fluxes of slow neutrons were encountered and a combination of three ionization chambers was used. These chambers were homogeneous or effectively so and were filled with acetylene, argon and boron trifluoride. A fourth chamber of tissue-like composition replaced the acetylene chamber for some measurements. The radiation sensitivities of these chambers are calculated below. The consideration of such matters as the attenuation of radiation in the chamber walls, and the energy dissipation per ion pair in the gas fillings has been left to a later stage as this seemed to improve the clarity of the presentation.

2. INTERACTION OF NEUTRONS WITH LIGHT ELEMENTS

When a beam of fast neutrons passes through matter, some of the neutrons will lose energy when they are scattered at elastic collisions with atomic nuclei. At a single collision, the average energy lost by the neutron will be very nearly $2A_i\epsilon/(1+A_i)^2$ (Chap. II, §3 (i), p. 32), where A_i is the atomic weight of the atom involved and ϵ the neutron energy before the collision. After a large number of such encounters, the energy of a neutron will tend towards the value $3kT/2$ where k is the Boltzmann constant and T the absolute temperature. At large depths in a medium one would expect that most of the neutrons would have this average energy, neglecting for the moment the possibility of capture. In practice, the cross section for capture generally increases with decreasing neutron velocity and some neutrons, mostly of low energy, will be captured in the medium. Neutrons may also be scattered inelastically when their energy is not less than the excitation energy of the nucleus which is struck.

The energy Q which is released when a neutron is captured can reappear in several forms. For instance, with thermal neutrons in the reaction $^1H(n,\gamma)^2D$, for which $Q = 2{\cdot}23$ MeV (Hornyak, Lauritsen, Morrison and Fowler, 1950), the energy is concentrated in a single gamma quantum, whilst in the nuclear reaction

$^{10}B\,(n,\alpha)^{7*}Li$ ($Q = 2{\cdot}79$ MeV) the α particle and excited $^{7*}Li$ recoil share 2·31 MeV, the rest appearing as a quantum of 0·478 MeV when the excited lithium nucleus goes to its ground state. When the product nucleus is radioactive, further energy Q' is set free later as a β particle (as in ^{14}C) or as a β particle and gamma ray, e.g. ^{28}Al. In general, if Q' is the radiation energy emitted by a radioactive product nucleus, the total energy set free is $Q+Q'+\epsilon$, where ϵ is the energy of the incident neutron. The term Q' may or may not be of significance depending upon the half-life of the radioactive nucleus and the time factor in the radiation effect under consideration.

When such reactions occur in a body of finite size, the average fraction of the energy $Q+Q'+\epsilon$ which is absorbed within it, depends upon its dimensions in relation to the ranges of the particles. For example, nearly all the energy carried by protons arising from the reaction $^{14}N(n,p)^{14}C$ in a body of the size of a mouse will be dissipated within it, whilst only a small fraction of the energy set free as gamma rays in the reaction $^{1}H(n,\gamma)^{2}D$ will be absorbed.

In the present work, neutrons were produced by fission in uranium (Chap. I, §8, p. 10). The energy spectrum of the neutrons reaching the irradiation spaces in the tanks can be considered as the sum of two continuous components, one of low energy with a peak in the neighbourhood of thermal energy (0·04 eV) and the other of high energy with a spectrum derived from the uranium fission spectrum modified by some degree of inelastic scattering (Chap. II, §7, (i), p. 38). We shall consider in detail the energy absorption in biological tissue and in the ionization chambers when they are irradiated by these neutrons.

The principal constituents of tissue are hydrogen, carbon, nitrogen and oxygen, the atomic percentages of which are respectively 62·8, 9·5, 1·35 and 25·7 ('Standard Man', p. 28). Other elements in tissue may be disregarded in so far as energy absorption is concerned. For the various ionization chambers the above elements and in addition boron, fluorine, magnesium, aluminium, argon and copper have to be considered.

The energy communicated to a tissue-like medium when it is exposed to neutrons from uranium fission arises almost entirely from elastic collisions, (mainly with neutrons of high energy), and from capture reactions, (mainly with neutrons of low energy for which the cross sections vary as $\epsilon^{-\frac{1}{2}}$). If the relative numbers of neutrons of high and low energy were known, the amounts of energy absorbed in tissue by the two processes could be calculated from a measurement of the ionization in a tissue chamber. The energy spectrum of the neutrons, however, was unknown, so it was necessary to measure the ionization current in two chambers, one containing hydrogen, which interacts primarily by elastic scattering, and the other an element such as boron, which has a very large capture cross section for low energy neutrons, the magnitude of this cross section being proportional to $\epsilon^{-\frac{1}{2}}$.

The relative quantities of energy absorbed in the tissue, acetylene and boron trifluoride chambers employed in this work over the energy range 1 eV to 10 MeV are shown in Fig. 6. It will be seen

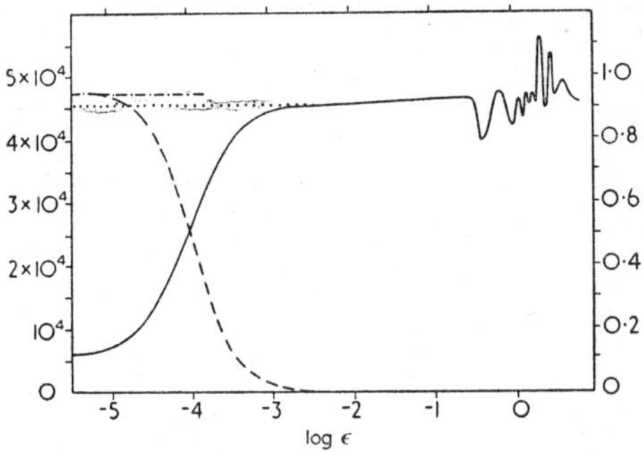

FIG. 6. Energy absorptions per gramme of gas in the acetylene and the boron trifluoride chambers relative to that in the tissue chamber as functions of neutron energy ϵ (MeV).

Ratio for C_2H_2 and tissue (right-hand scale)	total	————————
	scatter only	....
Ratio for BF_3 and tissue (left-hand scale)	total	– – – – – – – –
	capture only	– · – · – · – ·

that the total energy absorption in the boron trifluoride chamber (by neutron capture and scattering) is proportional to that in the tissue chamber for energies below 10 eV, whilst the total energy absorption in the acetylene chamber is approximately proportional to that in tissue for energies greater than 10^3 eV, except at the resonance peaks in the scattering cross sections for oxygen and carbon. Since the ionization in a chamber is proportional to the total energy absorbed within it, the observed ionization in the acetylene chamber, corrected for ionization by capture of low energy neutrons, will be a measure of the energy absorption by scattering in tissue. Similarly, the observed ionization in the boron trifluoride chamber after allowing for the ionization by recoil particles from elastic neutron collisions, will be a measure of the energy absorption by the capture reactions in tissue. For neutrons of energy less than 10 eV or greater than 10^3 eV, the energy absorption in the tissue chamber by both types of interaction can therefore be found by simultaneous measurements with the acetylene and boron trifluoride chambers. For energies between

10 eV and 10^3 eV, the interpretation of such measurements is not possible without a knowledge of the neutron energy spectrum, but in our experiment the number of neutrons with energies in this range was probably very small and their contribution to the total ionization in the acetylene and boron fluoride chambers was negligible. In terms of energy absorption this would imply that the spectrum can be considered as comprising a low energy group ($\epsilon < 10$ eV) and a high energy group ($\epsilon > 10^3$ eV) only. The writers have therefore adopted the following arbitrary convention based upon the mode of interaction of the neutrons with the gases of the ionization chambers. Neutrons which produce ionization in a particular chamber by capture reactions for which the cross sections are proportional to $\epsilon^{-\frac{1}{2}}$ are termed slow, whilst those which cause ionization in the chamber by elastic collisions or other nuclear reactions for which the cross sections are not proportional to $\epsilon^{-\frac{1}{2}}$ are termed fast. In practice, the other nuclear reactions can be neglected in tissue and in the ionization chambers used, as shown later.

3. ENERGY ABSORPTION DUE TO FAST NEUTRONS

(i) *Elastic Scattering of Fast Neutrons*

At a single elastic collision between a neutron of energy ϵ and an atom of a particular type denoted by the suffix i the energy transfer is

$$\frac{2A_i\epsilon}{(1+A_i)^2}(1-\cos\theta)$$

where A_i is the atomic weight of the atom and θ the angle of scattering of the neutron in centre of mass coordinates. At energies of the order of 1MeV the angular distribution of scattered neutrons in centre of mass coordinates is generally anisotropic, and the average energy ϵ_i exchanged per collision is given by

$$\epsilon_i = \frac{2A_i\epsilon}{(1+A_i)^2}K_i(\epsilon) \tag{1}$$

where

$$K_i(\epsilon) = \int_0^\pi \frac{\sigma_i(\theta, \epsilon)}{\sigma_i(\epsilon)}.(1-\cos\theta).2\pi\sin\theta\, d\theta \tag{2}$$

and $\sigma_i(\epsilon)$, $\sigma_i(\theta,\epsilon)$ are respectively the total and differential elastic scattering cross sections for neutrons of energy ϵ and atoms of type i. The scattering in hydrogen is exceptional, in that the value of $\sigma_i(\theta)$ is constant within ± 7 per cent at energies around 3 MeV

(Caplehorn and Rundle, 1951; Hamouda and Montmollin, 1952) and within ± 6 per cent at 14 MeV (Barschall, 1952). It has therefore been assumed that (n, p) scattering is strictly isotropic for neutrons from uranium fission so that $K_H = 1$ and the average energy of the recoil protons is $\epsilon/2$.

When a medium containing n_i atoms of type i per unit mass is exposed to a flux $N(\epsilon)\,d\epsilon$ of neutrons whose energies lie between ϵ and $\epsilon + d\epsilon$, the energy absorption per unit mass per unit time ${}_nE_i$ is given by

$$ {}_nE_i = \frac{2n_i A_i}{(1+A_i)^2} \int_0^\infty N(\epsilon) \, . \, \sigma_i(\epsilon) \, . \, K_i(\epsilon) \, . \, \epsilon \, d\epsilon \tag{3} $$

In media containing atoms of more than one type the total energy absorption is equal to the sum of the contributions by each. In the case of tissue ($H_{1 \cdot 00}C_{0 \cdot 15}N_{0 \cdot 02}O_{0 \cdot 41}$) and the hydrocarbon medium (CH) used in one of the chambers, the contribution by recoil protons, viz.:

$$ {}_nE_H = \tfrac{1}{2} n_H \int_0^\infty N(\epsilon) \, . \, \sigma_H(\epsilon) \, . \, \epsilon \, d\epsilon \tag{4} $$

accounts for most of the total energy absorption. The value of the fraction varies between relatively narrow limits except at the large resonance peaks in the elastic cross sections of oxygen (0·44, 1·00, 1·32 and 3·5 MeV) and carbon (2·9 and 3·5 MeV) (BNL-325). For neutrons whose energy spectrum is continuous over a wide energy range, the overall effect of these resonance peaks is small and does not depend sensitively on the form of the neutron spectrum (Table 2).

(ii) *Inelastic Scattering and Nuclear Reactions of Fast Neutrons*

Although there are several modes of interaction between fast neutrons and light nuclei, the cross sections of most of them are very small compared with the elastic scattering cross sections. The most important exceptions to this general rule are inelastic scattering at neutron energies well above threshold and particular reactions such as $^{14}N(n,p)^{14}C$ and $^{14}N(n, \alpha)^{11}B$ which have resonances in the energy range 0·5 to 2 MeV (BNL-325).

The inelastic scattering of neutrons with ^{12}C, ^{14}N and ^{16}O does not appear to have been investigated, but since the first excited levels of these nuclei are at 4·47, 2·3 and 6·05 MeV respectively (Hornyak *et al.*, 1950) and the threshold energies cannot be less than these values, it is unlikely that this process will contribute appreciably to energy deposition in biological tissues for the neutrons used in the present experiments (average energy 0·7 MeV, Chap. I, §11, p. 23).

The results quoted by Adair (1950) for the (n, p) and (n, α) reaction cross sections with nitrogen have been used to estimate the contribution to energy absorption by these processes relative to that by elastic scattering, assuming that the latter is isotropic in centre of mass coordinates. The energy communicated to tissue by nitrogen recoils is, however, so small compared with that by proton recoils (0·2 per cent), that the further refinement of allowing for these reactions in tissue becomes unnecessary.

4. ENERGY ABSORPTION DUE TO SLOW NEUTRONS

Consider a small element of a medium containing n_i atoms of type i per unit mass, exposed to a flux $N(\epsilon)\,\mathrm{d}\epsilon$ of neutrons of energy between ϵ and $\epsilon+\mathrm{d}\epsilon$. If ${}_a\sigma_i(\epsilon)$ is the absorption cross section for neutrons of energy ϵ in nuclei of type i and Q_i is the reaction energy, the energy ${}_sE$ set free in unit mass of the medium per second is given by

$$ {}_sE = \sum^{i} n_i \int_0^\infty (Q_i+\epsilon) N(\epsilon)\, {}_a\sigma_i(\epsilon)\, \mathrm{d}\epsilon. \tag{5} $$

When radioactive nuclei are produced, Q_i in this expression should be replaced by $Q_i+f_iQ'_i$ where Q'_i is the total energy emitted by the radioactive product nucleus. The quantity f_i is less than unity during the build up of the radioactivity and is equal to the ratio of the rate of decay of the radioactive nuclei to their rate of production. If the neutron irradiation is continued for a time which is long compared with the half life, f_i will tend towards unity.

The energy ${}_sE$ which is set free may not all be absorbed locally. For short-range particles such as protons or α particles the energy can be regarded as being completely absorbed except in the case of very small bodies, such as single biological cells, whose dimensions are comparable with the particle ranges. For the more penetrating β and γ radiation, the fraction of the energy which is absorbed will decrease as the size of the body in which it is produced diminishes. In such cases Q_i and Q'_i must be replaced by effective values.

When the absorption cross section for atoms of type i is proportional to $\epsilon^{-\frac{1}{2}}$ (e.g., boron, BNL-325) the energy released per unit mass per second is

$$ {}_sE = \sum^{i} n_i\, {}_a\sigma_i(\epsilon_T) \int_0^\infty (Q_i+\epsilon) N(\epsilon) \left(\frac{3kT}{2\epsilon}\right)^{\frac{1}{2}} \mathrm{d}\epsilon \tag{6} $$

where ${}_a\sigma_i(\epsilon_T)$ is the absorption cross section for neutrons of energy $(3kT/2)$. In most cases ϵ can be omitted from the term $(Q_i+\epsilon)$ in (6) without introducing an appreciable error. For example, the energy spectrum of neutrons in the irradiation tanks can be considered as the sum of two parts (Chap. II, §2, p. 29), a low energy component with a Maxwellian distribution ($\bar{\epsilon} = 3kT/2$) and a high energy component corresponding to the modified fission spectrum (Chap. II, §7 (i), p. 38). The rate of energy absorption in an element for which ${}_a\sigma_i(\epsilon)$ is proportional to $\epsilon^{-\frac{1}{2}}$ can then be written

$$ {}_sE_i = n_i\, {}_a\sigma_i(\epsilon_T) \left\{ Q_i S \left(\frac{6}{\pi}\right)^{\frac{1}{2}} + \left(\frac{3kT}{2}\right)^{\frac{1}{2}} N \left[(2Q_i+1)\, \mathrm{erf}\left(\frac{1}{\sqrt{2}}\right) + e^{-\frac{1}{2}} \right] \right\} \quad (7) $$

where S and N are the fluxes of the low energy and high energy components respectively and all energies are expressed in MeV. In fact $S/N > 0{\cdot}1$ (Tables 1 and 2 and values of n_i for tissue) whilst the coefficient of S in equation (7) exceeds that of N by the factor $1{\cdot}38\,.\,10^4 Q_i/(1{\cdot}80 + 2{\cdot}66 Q_i)$. The value of this factor for the reaction ${}^{10}B(n, \alpha)^7Li(Q_B = 2{\cdot}793$ MeV) is $4{\cdot}2\,.\,10^3$. Accordingly the simpler expression obtained by omitting ϵ from the term $(Q_i+\epsilon)$ in (6), viz.

$$ {}_sE_B = \sum^{i} n_i Q_i\, {}_a\sigma_i(\epsilon_T) \int_0^\infty N(\epsilon) \left(\frac{3kT}{2\epsilon}\right)^{\frac{1}{2}} d\epsilon \quad (8) $$

represents the rate of energy absorption by this reaction to an accuracy of 0·24 per cent or better.

For the elements hydrogen, nitrogen and argon, the absence of resonances in their total cross sections below 10^{-3} MeV (BNL-325) implies that their capture cross sections will be proportional to $\epsilon^{-\frac{1}{2}}$ when $\epsilon \ll 10^{-3}$ MeV. The capture cross sections of thermal neutrons in carbon (4·5 mb) and oxygen (< 0·2 mb) are very small, and there are no resonances. It has therefore been assumed that for elements in tissue and in the gases used in the ionization chambers, ${}_a\sigma_i(\epsilon)$ is proportional to $\epsilon^{-\frac{1}{2}}$. Since the effective values of Q_i and Q'_i for the reactions of low energy neutrons with H, C, N, O, normally greatly exceed thermal energies we may write ϵ for $(Q_i+\epsilon)$, so that

$$ {}_sE = {}_sE_B \cdot \frac{\sum^{i} n_i Q_i\, {}_a\sigma_i(\epsilon_T)}{n_B Q_B\, {}_a\sigma_B(\epsilon_T)} \quad (9) $$

in which ${}_sE_B$ can be found from ionization measurements with a boron chamber.

5. ENERGY ABSORPTION DUE TO GAMMA RAYS

The average energy of the gamma rays in the irradiation tanks has been found experimentally to be $0{\cdot}68 \pm 0{\cdot}08$ MeV (Chap. II, §15 (ii, c), p. 72). At such energies the only important mode of interaction with elements of low atomic number is Compton scattering. Even for magnesium the photoelectric absorption cross section per electron, τ, is less than one per cent of the electronic cross section σ_a associated with the energy absorption by recoil electrons, whilst pair production at the high energy tail of the spectrum is still comparatively unimportant. This is evident from a rough calculation. Thus, if one assumes, in the absence of detailed knowledge of the spectrum, that 20 per cent of all photons have an energy of 3 MeV, pair production in magnesium would account for one per cent of the total energy absorption (Davisson and Evans, 1952). Photonuclear reactions are of no practical consequence for the present purpose as their cross sections are only ~ 1 mb or less, whilst the value of the Compton scattering coefficient per electron σ_a is about 100 mb.

Thus for the light elements ($Z = 1$ to $Z = 12$) the rate of energy absorption, ${}_{\gamma}E$, in a medium containing n_i atoms of type i per unit mass is

$$ {}_{\gamma}E = G\bar{\sigma}_a \sum^{i} n_i Z_i \qquad (10) $$

where G is the energy flux of gamma radiation and $\bar{\sigma}_a$ is the average electronic cross section associated with energy transfer to recoil electrons. The latter is given by

$$ \bar{\sigma}_a = \frac{\int_0^\infty N(\nu) h\nu \sigma_a \, d\nu}{\int_0^\infty N(\nu) h\nu \, d\nu} \qquad (11) $$

$N(\nu)\,d\nu$ being the number of photons of frequency between ν and $\nu + d\nu$ and h Planck's constant.

6. THE PRINCIPLE OF THE METHOD OF MEASUREMENT OF FAST NEUTRON DOSE

We have measured the radiation doses due to fast neutrons from uranium fission and to the gamma rays and slow neutrons which accompany them by the ionization method (Gray, 1929, 1936, 1944). This method is based on the relation between the energy absorption in an irradiated medium and the ionization in a small gas-filled cavity within it. If the rate of energy absorption per unit mass of the medium is E and the rate of ionization per unit mass of gas is J, Gray showed that

$$E = \rho WJ \tag{12}$$

where ρ is the ratio of the mass stopping powers of the medium and of the gas for the secondary ionizing particles generated, and W is the average energy expended in the production of one pair of ions in the gas. When the atomic composition of the gas differs from that of the medium, this relation is only true if the dimensions of the cavity are small compared with the range in the gas of the secondary particles. When the atomic compositions are identical it holds for a cavity of any size, provided that the primary radiation distribution is uniform over the dimensions of the chamber. Thus one can estimate the energy absorption in irradiated tissue by measuring the ionization in a chamber whose walls are of tissue-like material, either by using a small chamber filled with air or other suitable gas or by using one of any convenient size filled with gas whose atomic composition is the same as that of the walls. Chambers of the latter type are usually termed homogeneous.

Consider an ionization chamber exposed to fast neutrons, slow neutrons and gamma rays. Suppose that the wall thickness of the chamber exceeds the range of the fastest secondary ionizing particles and that p_1, q_1 and r_1 are the small fractional losses in the wall of gamma ray energy flux, fast neutron energy flux and slow neutron flux respectively. The ionization rate, i.e. the total number, J_1, of ion pairs per unit mass of gas per second can be written in the form

$$J_1 = (1-p_1)a_{1\gamma}D+(1-q_1)b_{1n}D+(1-r_1)c_1S \tag{13}$$

where ${}_\gamma D$, ${}_n D$ are respectively the dosage rates due to gamma radiation and fast neutrons, S is the flux of slow neutrons and a_1, b_1 and c_1 are numerical constants, the values of which depend upon the atomic composition of the chamber and the energies of the radiations.

Suppose now that two other chambers of different composition are exposed simultaneously with the first in the same radiation field. The ionization rates in these chambers J_2 and J_3 can be expressed in the same form as J_1 and from the three equations together, ${}_\gamma D$, ${}_n D$ and S can be written in terms of J_1, J_2, J_3 and a_1, b_1, c_1; p_1, q_1, r_1; .... The methods of evaluating a_1, b_1, c_1 ... are described first and those for p_1, q_1, r_1 ... afterwards (Chap. II, §10, p. 49).

7. IONIZATION DOSE RELATIONS FOR FAST NEUTRONS

(i) *Homogeneous Acetylene and Tissue Chambers*

The ionization rate in a homogeneous chamber exposed to fast neutrons is equal to the rate of energy absorption by recoil particles in the gas divided by the average energy loss per ion pair produced. The contribution to the energy absorption by recoil protons can be calculated accurately for neutrons of a given energy since (n, p) scattering is isotropic in centre of mass coordinates and its cross section is well known. Experimental data on the total elastic cross sections of carbon, nitrogen and oxygen are adequate in the energy range of interest, but the angular distributions of neutrons scattered by these nuclei have been investigated at a very few neutron energies only (BNL-325). For example, the only published results for oxygen are for neutron energies of 2·0, 2·9 and 3·44 MeV where the deviations from isotropic scattering in centre of mass coordinates are so large that energy absorption in this element may be as small as one-half of that calculated on the assumption of isotropic scattering. A similar factor is indicated by the data for carbon at 2·7 MeV and some higher energies, but below 1·5 MeV the deviations from isotropic scattering appear to be unimportant. In the absence of more complete information over a much wider range of energies, the present calculations have been made assuming isotropic scattering for neutrons of all energies in elastic collisions with carbon, nitrogen and oxygen nuclei.

The rate of energy absorption per unit mass in a medium composed of atoms of type i, equation (3), can then be written (putting $K_i = 1$)

$$_nE_i = \frac{2A_i}{(1+A_i)^2} \int_0^\infty N(\epsilon)\sigma_i(\epsilon) \, . \, \epsilon \, d\epsilon. \tag{14}$$

The integral in this expression has been evaluated graphically for the elements hydrogen, carbon, nitrogen and oxygen using the cross sections given in report BNL-325. The calculations were made for

(1) a neutron spectrum $N(\epsilon) = N.(2/e\pi)^{\frac{1}{2}} e^{-\epsilon} \sinh(2\epsilon)^{\frac{1}{2}}$ corresponding to prompt neutrons of energy ϵ MeV from the fission of ^{235}U (Watt, 1952), N being the total flux and $(2/e\pi)^{\frac{1}{2}}$ the normalizing factor.

(2) a distribution $N(\epsilon) = N.(8/e\pi)^{\frac{1}{2}} e^{-2\epsilon} \sinh(4\epsilon)^{\frac{1}{2}}$ which for convenience will be termed the modified fission spectrum and which represents the spectrum of neutrons emerging from the lead absorbers over the uranium (Chap. I, §9, p. 12) on the

arbitrary assumption that the energies of all neutrons are halved by inelastic (and elastic) collisions in their passage through the lead, and

(3) neutrons of 0·7 MeV, this being the average energy as determined by experiment (Chapter I, §11, p. 23).

The numerical values of the energy absorption per atom per neutron per cm², viz. ${}_nE_i/Nn_i$ for hydrogen, carbon, nitrogen and oxygen for each of these three neutron spectra are recorded in Table 2.

TABLE 2

Energy absorption (eV . 10^{-18}) per atom per neutron per cm² for each of the three neutron energy distributions; data for hydrogen, carbon, nitrogen, and oxygen

Atom	(1) Fission spectrum	(2) Modified fission spectrum	(3) 0·7 MeV
H	2·61	1·926	1·79
C	0·545	0·338	0·296
N	0·471	0·256	0·211
O	0·468	0·317	0·229

Now from the definition of the rad the rate of energy absorption (in electron volts/gramme/second) in tissue ($H_{1\cdot00}C_{0\cdot15}N_{0\cdot02}O_{0\cdot41}$) exposed to a fast neutron dosage rate of ${}_nD$ rads/hour is given by

$$\sum^{\text{tissue}} {}_nE_i = \frac{100\,.\,6{\cdot}24\,.\,10^{11}}{3600}\,{}_nD = 1{\cdot}733\,.\,10^{10}\,{}_nD. \qquad (15)$$

The coefficient b (equation (13)) for a homogeneous chamber can therefore be written (when $q = 0$)

$$b = \frac{{}_nJ}{{}_nD} = \frac{\overset{\text{gas}}{\Sigma}\,{}_nE_i}{W\,{}_nD} = \frac{\overset{\text{gas}}{\Sigma}\,{}_nE_i\,.\,1{\cdot}733\,.\,10^{10}}{\underset{}{\overset{\text{tissue}}{\Sigma}}\,{}_nE_i \quad W} \qquad (16)$$

where $\overset{\text{gas}}{\Sigma}\,{}_nE_i$ is the rate of energy absorption per gramme of gas in the chamber and W is the average energy (in eV) expended by the neutron recoils in producing one pair of ions in the gas.

The values of $\overset{\text{tissue}}{\Sigma}\,{}_nE_i$ and of $\overset{\text{gas}}{\Sigma}\,{}_nE_i$ for the acetylene and tissue chambers have been found from the data in Table 2 by inserting the appropriate values of n_i. For the neutron spectra (1), (2) and (3) the quantity $\overset{\text{tissue}}{\Sigma}\,{}_nE_i$ has the values $1{\cdot}727\,.\,10^5$, $1{\cdot}261\,.\,10^5$ and $1{\cdot}150\,.\,10^5$ eV/g/n/cm²/sec respectively and the products bW for the chambers have the values given in Table 3. It will be noted that the rate of energy absorption in the gas of the tissue chamber was about 8 per

TABLE 3

The rates of energy absorption, bW(eV g^{-1} sec^{-1} . 10^{+10}) in the gas fillings of the homogeneous acetylene and tissue chambers for each of the three neutron energy distributions and a dose rate of 1 *rad* hr^{-1}

Chamber	(1) Fission spectrum	(2) Modified fission spectrum	(3) 0·7 MeV
Acetylene	1·452	1·430	1·440
Tissue†	1·600	1·598	1·595

† Although not strictly homogeneous, the walls and gas of this chamber were of almost identical composition (Chap. II, § 14 (i), p. 61).

cent smaller than in standard tissue (equation 15), owing to a small difference in atomic composition. If required, the data in Table 3 (and Table 4, below) can be expressed in terms of fast neutron flux instead of dose rate, using a conversion factor derived from the above values of $\overset{\text{tissue}}{\Sigma_n} E_i$ in conjunction with equation (15).

No experimental measurements of the energy expenditure per ion pair for neutron recoils in the gas fillings of our chambers have been made so the appropriate values of *W* have been inferred from the published data for other particles, mainly alphas. Two alternative values of *W* have been derived (Chap. II, §16 (v), p. 80), one on the assumption that *W* is actually constant for all ionizing particles in a given gas and the other on the assumption that it is a function of the type and speed of the particle. These values of *W* are given in Table 4 for the gas-fillings of the acetylene and tissue chambers

TABLE 4

Ionization rate, b, (*ions* sec^{-1} g^{-1} . 10^{+8}) *in the gases of the acetylene and tissue chambers for each of the three neutron energy distributions and a dose rate of* 1 *rad* hr^{-1}

Chamber	Energy/ion pair (*W*) assumed to be	(1) Fission spectrum		(2) Modified fission spectrum		(3) 0·7 MeV	
		W(eV)	*b*	*W*(eV)	*b*	*W*(eV)	*b*
Acetylene	Constant	27·5	5·28	27·5	5·20	27·5	5·23
	Variable	28·9	5·02	29·5	4·85	29·6	4·87
Tissue	Constant	34·5	4·63	34·5	4·62	34·5	4·61
	Variable	36·1	4·42	36·8	4·34	37·0	4·31

together with the corresponding values of b. The dose rates given in Table 1 were calculated using values of b for modified fission neutrons and for W varying with particle speed. Earlier estimates of b based on very scanty data for the energy per ion pair in acetylene gave dose rates 20 per cent higher (Neary, Munson and Mole, 1953).

(ii) *Non-Homogeneous Chambers*

There are two non-homogeneous chambers for which the values of b are required, viz magnesium-argon and copper-boron trifluoride. For each of these chambers the ranges of recoil nuclei are small compared with the dimensions of the gas volume. One would therefore expect that the ionization in either chamber would be very closely similar to that in a homogeneous chamber with the same gas filling. The magnitude of the small wall effect can be found in the following way.

Suppose, for simplicity, that all recoils originating in the walls have energy ϵ_w and those produced in the gas ϵ_g. If the neutron scattering cross sections are denoted by σ_w, σ_g for these two types of atom and n_w, n_g are the numbers of atoms per unit mass in the wall and gas, the ionization per unit mass per second per unit flux in the bulk of the gas is

$$J_g = \frac{\epsilon_g n_g \sigma_g}{W_g} \tag{17}$$

whilst the ionization in a very small gas-filled cavity in the wall is given by

$$J_w = \frac{\epsilon_w n_w \sigma_w}{W_w} \frac{n_g s_g}{n_w s_w} \tag{18}$$

where W_g is the average energy expended by the gas recoils in producing one pair of ions, W_w the corresponding quantity for the wall recoils and s_w, s_g are respectively the atomic stopping powers of the wall and gas for recoils generated in the wall.

The ionization at the surface of the chamber wall will be $\frac{1}{2}(J_g+J_w)$ and if the ionization is assumed to change linearly with distance from the wall until it reaches the value J_g at a distance from the wall equal to the range, the average ionization within this thin layer of gas is $\frac{1}{2}[\frac{1}{2}(J_w+J_g)+J_g]$ which exceeds that in a homogeneous chamber by $\frac{1}{4}(J_w-J_g)$. The average ionization per unit mass per second in the whole gas is therefore greater than J_g by the factor F where

$$F = 1+\frac{AR}{4V}\left(\frac{J_w}{J_g}-1\right) \tag{19}$$

where A is the superficial area of the chamber walls, V the total gas volume and R is the range in the gas of the wall recoils.

A more realistic calculation of the ionization due to wall recoils can be made if one assumes that the range of recoils of a given type in the gas is proportional to (energy)^m. This leads to a new factor

$$F' = 1+\frac{ARm}{4V(1+m)}\left(\frac{J_w}{J_g}-\frac{R'}{R}\right) \tag{20}$$

where R' is the range in the gas of the gas recoils.

From a recent investigation by Mills (1952), who used a low-pressure cloud chamber, it appears that for energies $\sim 0{\cdot}1$ MeV, the ranges of protons, α particles and oxygen ions in cm of air are approximately equal to $0{\cdot}82\times(A_i)^{-1/3}$ (energy)$^{2/3}$, where A_i is the atomic weight of the particle (0 = 16) and its energy is expressed in MeV. Assuming that this expression also applies to the low energy recoils in the ionization chambers, one can calculate their ranges in air and thence find R and R' using the stopping power data of Aron, Hoffman and Williams (1949). When the energies of the recoils are taken as $2A_i/(1+A_i)^2$ MeV, corresponding to a neutron energy of 1 MeV, and the corresponding values of R and R' are inserted in equation (20) together with the values of A, V and

$$\frac{J_w}{J_g}\left(=\frac{E_w}{E_g}\cdot\frac{\sigma_w}{\sigma_g}\cdot\frac{s_g}{s_w}\cdot\frac{W_g}{W_w}\right),$$

the factor F' is found to be $1{\cdot}014$ for the magnesium-argon chamber, and $0{\cdot}997$ for the copper-boron trifluoride chamber. It is therefore clear that both chambers may be treated as homogeneous or 'free gas' chambers. The quantities ${}_nE_i/Nn_i$, bW and b were calculated for argon and boron trifluoride by the method described above for the gases of the acetylene and tissue chambers. The results are given in Tables 5, 6 and 7. Since no measurements of the scattering cross section of argon have been reported at neutron energies greater than $1{\cdot}1$ MeV, the calculations were made on the plausible assumption that the cross section decreased linearly from $1{\cdot}8$ barn at $1{\cdot}1$ MeV to $0{\cdot}9$ barn at 10 MeV. However, any error introduced in this way has a very small overall effect upon the accuracy of the final estimates of fast neutron and gamma ray dose rates.

TABLE 5

Energy absorption ($eV . 10^{-18}$) per atom per neutron per cm^2 for each of the three neutron energy distributions; data for boron, fluorine, and argon

Atom	(1) Fission spectrum	(2) Modified fission spectrum	(3) 0·7 MeV
B	0·580	0·355	0·402
F	0·450	0·298	0·226
A	0·146	0·080	0·035

TABLE 6

The rates of energy absorption, bW($eV\ g^{-1}\ sec^{-1} . 10^{+10}$) in the gas fillings of the copper-boron trifluoride and magnesium-argon chambers, for each of the three neutron energy distributions and a dose rate of 1 *rad hr*$^{-1}$

Chamber	(1) Fission spectrum	(2) Modified fission spectrum	(3) 0·7 MeV
Cu–BF_3	0·172	0·153	0·145
Mg–A	0·022	0·017	0·008

TABLE 7

Ionization rate, b, (ions $sec^{-1}\ g^{-1} . 10^{+8}$) in the gases of the copper-boron trifluoride and magnesium-argon chambers for each of the three neutron energy distributions and a dose rate of 1 *rad hr*$^{-1}$

Chamber	Energy/ion pair (W) assumed to be	(1) Fission spectrum		(2) Modified fission spectrum		(3) 0·7 MeV	
		W(eV)	b	W(eV)	b	W(eV)	b
Cu–BF_3	Constant	36·1	0·476	36·1	0·424	36·1	0·400
	Variable	48·2	0·367	57·1	0·268	59·2	0·245
Mg–A	Constant	26·3	0·084	26·3	0·063	26·3	0·030

8. IONIZATION FLUX RELATIONS FOR SLOW NEUTRONS

The ionization currents in the chambers caused by slow neutrons in the experimental tanks were small compared with those produced by fast neutrons and gamma rays, except in the case of the boron trifluoride chamber. However, it seemed worth while to calculate the response of each chamber with reasonable accuracy, in order to deal with the more general problem.

The calculation of the ionization currents to be expected per unit neutron flux has been carried out on the assumption that the energy distribution of the slow neutrons was Maxwellian with a mean energy of $3kT/2$, T being taken as 293°K. The cross sections were assumed to vary inversely as the neutron velocity and hence the effective cross section was $\sqrt{(6/\pi)}$ times that at the velocity corresponding to an energy $3kT/2$. If in fact the distribution was not Maxwellian the numerical factor relating ionization to flux will be in error, but the error will be the same for all chambers (Chap. II, §4, p. 34). Thus, although these calculations will not permit an estimate of absolute neutron flux from the observed ionization in the boron trifluoride chamber, they will give the ionization to be expected in another chamber irradiated by the same slow neutrons and this is the information required for the present purpose.

Data on the reaction cross sections and the reaction products have been taken from BNL-325 and the tables of Hollander, Perlman and Seaborg (1953) respectively.

(i) *Boron Trifluoride Chamber*

The ionization current in the boron trifluoride chamber under slow neutron irradiation is due almost entirely to the α particles and ^{7}Li recoils from the $^{10}B(n, \alpha)^7Li$ reaction with very small contributions due to gamma rays from those ^{7}Li nuclei formed in an excited state (0·03 per cent) and beta rays from ^{66}Cu(0·01 per cent) produced in the chamber walls (Appendix, p. 84).

In order to calculate the ionization due to the α particles and ^{7}Li recoils it is necessary to know the approximate ranges of these particles in the gas. Three independent estimates of the molecular stopping power of boron trifluoride relative to air have been derived: the first, 2·28 from the tables given by Livingston and Bethe (1937) for 4·66 MeV α particles, the second, 1·96 from the results of Hatfield, Lockenitz and Colby (1949) for ^{210}Po α particles and the third, 2·12 from Warshaw's (1949) data for 0·5 MeV protons. If one assumes the value 2·1 for this ratio, the ranges of a 1·48 MeV α particle and a 0·86 MeV ^{7}Li recoil (the weighted means for the ground and excited states of the ^{7}Li nucleus) are 0·34 and 0·18 cm respectively, according to the range-energy relation given above (Chap. II, §7 (ii), p. 42). Since these ranges are small compared with the inter-electrode spacing, the ionization may be calculated on the assumption that the chamber is effectively a free gas chamber. A small correction may then be applied (as in Chap. II, §7, (ii), p. 41), to allow for the wall effect. Since J_w/J_g is negligible, the ionization due to each type of particle is equal to that in a gas-walled boron trifluoride chamber multiplied by the factor $[1-(AR'/4V)(m)/(m+1)]$, equation (20). Putting $m = 2/3$ and $A/V = 1$ cm, this factor is 0·960 for the α particle and 0·977 for the ^{7}Li. The ionization rates per unit flux due to α particles and ^{7}Li recoils were calculated from equation (8) and were found to be $3{\cdot}12 . 10^6$ and $1{\cdot}82 . 10^6$ ions g^{-1} sec^{-1} respectively in free boron trifluoride, taking $W = 36{\cdot}1$ eV for both particles (Table 18). When the wall correction factors were applied the total ionization rate was $4{\cdot}76 . 10^6$ ions g^{-1} sec^{-1} per unit flux of slow neutrons. Alternatively, if one assumes that for boron trifluoride W is dependent upon the initial speed of the particle (Chap. II, §16 (iv), p. 78) with $\mu = 0{\cdot}23$ (Appendix, p. 84), the total ionization rate is found to be $4{\cdot}42 . 10^6$ ions g^{-1} sec^{-1} per unit flux.

(ii) *Magnesium-Argon Chamber*

Magnesium has quite small slow neutron absorption and activation cross sections, so that the energy released as beta and gamma radiation in the wall gives rise to very small ionization currents with the slow neutron fluxes encountered in the present experiments.

The actual ionization currents to be expected from the various slow neutron reactions have been estimated using formulae given in the Appendix (p. 84). It was found that the ionization rate in the argon-filled magnesium chamber exposed to unit flux of slow neutrons was 10·6 ions g^{-1} sec^{-1}. This is the sum of contributions due to

(a) beta radiation from ^{27}Mg (2·2 ions g^{-1} sec^{-1})
(b) beta radiation from ^{41}A (1·7 ions g^{-1} sec^{-1})
(c) gamma radiation from ^{27}Mg (1·1 ions g^{-1} sec^{-1})
(d) gamma radiation from capture in ^{24}Mg, ^{25}Mg and ^{26}Mg (5·1 ions g^{-1} sec^{-1})
(e) gamma radiation from neutron absorption in Zn and Cu isotopes of external brass members (0·5 ions g^{-1} sec^{-1})

(iii) *Acetylene Chamber*

The largest source of ionization in the acetylene chamber exposed to slow neutrons is beta radiation from ^{28}Al formed by neutron capture in the outer aluminium sheath of this chamber. In the absence of the CH lining it has been calculated that this would lead to an ionization rate of 250 ions g^{-1} sec^{-1} in unit neutron flux (Appendix, p. 85). From the results of Gray (1936) the stopping power of the 0·24 g cm^{-2} of lining is equivalent to 0·10 cm of aluminium. The thickness of aluminium transmitting 50 per cent of ^{28}Al beta rays of 2·7 MeV maximum energy is 0·13 cm (*Science and Engineering of Nuclear Power*, Vol. 1, 1947) and according to Behrens (1948) the fraction transmitted through 0·10 cm aluminium is 57 per cent. One would therefore expect an ionization of 138 ions g^{-1} sec^{-1} from unit flux of slow neutrons from this source. Other sources of ionization are

(1) Gamma radiation produced in the lining by $^{1}H(n, \gamma)^{2}D$ (14 ions g^{-1} sec^{-1})
(2) Gamma radiation from ^{28}Al (7 ions g^{-1} sec^{-1})
(3) Capture gamma rays in ^{27}Al (15 ions g^{-1} sec^{-1})
(4) Gamma radiation from the brass components of the chamber (1 ion g^{-1} sec^{-1})

Thus the total ionization from all sources is 175 ions g^{-1} sec^{-1} in unit flux of slow neutrons.

For the second acetylene chamber (Chap. II, §14 (i), p. 59), in which all aluminium parts were replaced by magnesium, the ionization rate was 21 ions g^{-1} sec^{-1} per unit neutron flux. This was the sum of contributions from

(1) Gamma radiation from ^{27}Mg and from neutron capture in ^{24}Mg, ^{25}Mg and ^{26}Mg (3 ions g^{-1} sec^{-1})
(2) Gamma radiation from neutron capture in the CH lining (14 ions g^{-1} sec^{-1})
(3) Gamma radiation from the magnesium and 'Perspex' parts at one end of the chamber (4 ions g^{-1} sec^{-1})

(iv) *Tissue Chamber*

The slow neutron reactions leading to ionization in the tissue chamber are:

(1) $^{1}H(n, \gamma)^{2}D$ in the chamber wall (which gives rise to 35 ions g^{-1} sec^{-1} per unit flux of neutrons)
(2) $^{14}N\ (n, p)\ ^{14}C$ (66 ions g^{-1} sec^{-1})
(3) Gamma radiation from the brass components of the chamber (6 ions g^{-1} sec^{-1})

The total ionization in unit flux of thermal neutrons is thus 107 ions g^{-1} sec^{-1}.

(v) *Relative Ionizations by Fast and Slow Neutrons*

Data on the thermal fluxes in the irradiation tanks given in Table 1, together with the values of the coefficients c calculated above, give directly the number of ions produced per gramme of gas in each of the various chambers. This number is compared with the corresponding numbers of ions produced by fast neutrons and gamma rays in Table 8.

In view of the relatively small magnitude of the ionization currents

TABLE 8

Fraction of total ionization current due to slow neutrons

Tank	Shutter	Chamber	Fraction (%)
MAX	Open	$CH–C_2H_2$	0·74
		Mg–A	0·32
	Closed	$CH–C_2H_2$	0·35
		Mg–A	0·04
MED	Open	$CH–C_2H_2$	1·56
		Mg–A	0·24
	Closed	$CH–C_2H_2$	0·30
		Mg–A	0·03
MIN	Open	$CH–C_2H_2$	1·16
		Mg–A	0·12
	Closed	$CH–C_2H_2$	0·16
		Mg–A	0·02

in the acetylene, magnesium-argon and tissue chambers produced by slow neutrons in the irradiation tanks, it was thought that the values of the coefficients c estimated above were sufficiently precise. If however the slow neutron flux had been larger by an order of magnitude it would have been desirable to determine the values of c experimentally.

9. IONIZATION DOSE RELATIONS FOR GAMMA RAYS

We are primarily concerned with the ionization in chambers composed of light elements (acetylene, tissue and magnesium chambers) when they are exposed to gamma radiation in the experimental tanks and also to radium gamma rays. With light elements ($1 < Z < 12$) and gamma rays of energy between 0·4 and 1·8 MeV, the photoelectric and pair production coefficients per atom are both less than one per cent of the scattering absorption coefficient $Z\bar{\sigma}_a$, so that the energy absorption per gramme in the wall of one of the chambers containing n_w atoms per gramme of atomic number Z_w is $G\bar{\sigma}_a n_w Z_w$ per sec. (equation 10) with an error of one per cent or less. If the chamber is filled with a gas composed of n_g atoms per gramme of atomic number Z_g and the electronic stopping powers of the atoms in the gas and wall are respectively s_g and s_w per electron, the ratio of the mass stopping powers of the wall and gas is $(n_w Z_w s_w)/(n_g Z_g s_g)$, and from equation (12) the ionization rate in the gas can be written,

$$_{\gamma}J = \frac{G\bar{\sigma}_a n_g Z_g s_g}{W_g s_w} \tag{21}$$

where W_g is the average energy expended by secondary electrons in producing one ion pair. When the gas contains molecules of more than one type and when the number of molecules of each type which are ionized is unaffected by the presence of other types (Munson unpublished), the factor $n_g Z_g s_g / W_g$ in equation (21) should be replaced by

$$\overset{g}{\Sigma}\, n_g Z_g s_g / W_g$$

If also the wall contains atoms of more than one kind the ionization rate becomes

$$_{\gamma}J = G\bar{\sigma}_a(\overset{w}{\Sigma} n_w Z_w)\frac{\overset{g}{\Sigma}\, n_g Z_g s_g / W_g}{\overset{w}{\Sigma}\, n_w Z_w s_w} \tag{22}$$

From the definition of the roentgen (r) the gamma dose rate $_{\gamma}D$ in r/hour is given by

$$_{\gamma}D = \frac{3600 G\bar{\sigma}_a}{W_{\text{air}}} \overset{\text{air}}{\Sigma}\, n_g Z_g \tag{23}$$

which, on inserting the numerical values of n_g, Z_g for air, yields

$$G\bar{\sigma}_a = 1{\cdot}49 \, . \, 10^{-15}\, {}_{\gamma}D W_{\text{air}} \tag{24}$$

From (22) and (24) it follows that the coefficient a in equation (13) can be written

$$a = \frac{_{\gamma}J}{_{\gamma}D} = 1{\cdot}49 \, . \, 10^{-15}\, W_{\text{air}}(\overset{w}{\Sigma}\, n_w Z_w)\frac{\overset{g}{\Sigma}\, n_g Z_g s_g / W_g}{\overset{w}{\Sigma}\, n_w Z_w s_w} \tag{25}$$

when absorption of gamma radiation in the wall is neglected ($p = 0$). Using this expression values of a have been calculated for each of the chambers with the results given in Table 9. In the case of the copper-boron trifluoride chamber, equation (25) will give a value of a too

TABLE 9

Ionization rates, a, (ions sec^{-1} g^{-1} . 10^{-8}) in the various chambers exposed to gamma rays of energy 0·68 *MeV at a dose rate of* 1 *r hr^{-1}*

Chamber	s_g/s_w	W_{air}/W_g	a
Mg–A	0·96	1·29	5·02
Acetylene	1·00	1·32	6·31
Cu–BF_3	1·12	0·98	4·92
Tissue	1·00	1·06	5·18

low by approximately five per cent because of a contribution by photoelectric absorption, so the figure has been corrected by this amount.

The stopping power ratios were taken from the experimental results of Gray (1936) and values of W_{air}/W_g from a number of sources (Chap. II, §16, p. 72). In the special case where gamma rays only are present, the necessity for calculating a may be obviated by using a known gamma ray dose rate to calibrate the chamber.

10. ATTENUATION OF RADIATIONS IN THE CHAMBER WALLS

The values of the coefficients a, b, c, give the relation between dose rate and ionization chamber current only when each type of radiation suffers negligible absorption in the walls of the chambers. Wall absorption, however, is generally appreciable, and the necessary correction factors have been estimated theoretically and experimentally.

Since gamma rays and neutrons produce ionization indirectly through the agency of secondary particles, a substantial part of the ionization in a gas cavity may be due to those secondary particles produced in the wall. The wall thickness normally used is comparable to the range of the secondary particles, but a large proportion of the secondaries entering the cavity comes from a thin inside shell of the wall. It is appropriate in such cases to allow for attenuation of the primary radiation in the full wall-thickness. Since the primary radiation and its energy are not completely absorbed when a gamma quantum suffers a Compton collision or a fast neutron an elastic collision, effective cross sections for these processes, σ_a and $(2A_i\sigma_i)/(1+A_i)^2$ respectively, have been used. The particular case of the attenuation of gamma rays in the cylindrical walls of an ionization chamber is discussed below (Chap. II, §15 (ii, a), p. 67), and results embodied in formulae (43) and (44) are applicable also to the attenuation of fast and slow neutrons. With slow neutrons however, the secondary radiation produced in the wall may include gamma rays, and the observed ionization is not related in any simple manner to the attenuation of the primary radiation in the wall. Each case must be considered individually, and the attenuation factors for slow neutrons given below in Table 11 represent the overall corrections for particular chambers only.

In Table 10 the results of calculations and experimental measurements are given for attenuating sleeves of celluloid and aluminium. The latter were made to fit closely around the acetylene and magnesium-argon chambers which were exposed to the radiations in the

MAXIMUM tank (36·4 m rads/hr of fast neutrons, 6·95 mr/hr of gamma rays; the thermal neutrons may be neglected, see Table 8). The calculated attenuation factors for the fast neutrons and for the gamma rays are given in the second and third columns, where the values corresponding to the two assumed angular distributions of secondary ionizing particles, (i) isotropic emission, formula (43), and (ii) forward emission, formula (44), appear side by side. In calculating the attenuation for the mixed radiations $(n+\gamma)$, the averages of the factors for fast neutrons and gamma rays separately have been used, weighting these average values by the chamber sensitivity and dose rates.

TABLE 10

Calculated and observed percentage attenuation of fast neutrons and gamma rays in celluloid and aluminium sleeves

Sleeve	n only (calculated) (i)	(ii)	γ only (calculated) (i)	(ii)	Acetylene chamber $(n+\gamma)$ calc.	obs.	Magnesium chamber $(n+\gamma)$ calc.	obs.
Celluloid (4·0 mm)	5·3	4·8	2·5	2·3	5·0	4·85	2·6	2·3
Aluminium (3·2 mm)	0·25	0·25	3·5	3·4	0·8	0·8	3·3	2·8

There is satisfactory agreement between the observed and calculated attenuation factors for the mixed radiation in these two sleeves, so that the use of the same formulae for calculating losses in the walls of all the chambers seems justified. Table 11 contains the results of these calculations. Those for fast neutrons and gamma rays were derived using the average of the two attenuation factors

TABLE 11

Calculated percentage attenuation of fast neutrons, gamma rays and slow neutrons in the walls of the chambers

Chamber	Fast neutrons	Gamma rays	Slow neutrons
Magnesium-argon	1·5	3·0	0·1
Acetylene	4·3	2·9	0·4
Copper-boron trifluoride	0·1	1·7	1·8
Tissue	7·2	2·2	0·8

(43) and (44), whilst for slow neutrons the appropriate factor was given by formula (43) since in this case the secondary radiations were distributed isotropically.

11. EXPRESSIONS FOR FAST NEUTRON AND GAMMA RAY DOSE RATES AND FOR SLOW NEUTRON FLUX

The observed current from an ionization chamber can be expressed as the product of the ionization rate per gramme of gas and a numerical factor. This factor is proportional to chamber volume (at constant gas temperature and pressure) and the sensitivity of the current measuring system. Thus if H_1 denotes the value of the factor for chamber 1 and J_1 and M_1 are respectively the ionization rate and current reading (in arbitrary units) with this chamber $J_1 = M_1/H_1$. When chamber 1 is calibrated by exposure to gamma rays at a dose rate of d_1 r/hr (giving a reading ${}_cM_1$), the ionization rate ${}_cJ_1$ is, according to equation (13)

$${}_cJ_1 = (1-p_1)a_1d_1 \tag{26}$$

where p_1 is the fractional attenuation in the chamber wall of gamma rays from the calibration source and a_1 is the ionization rate corresponding to unit dose rate within the chamber gas. But

$${}_cJ_1 = \frac{{}_cM_1}{H_1} \tag{27}$$

so that

$$J_1 = \frac{M_1}{H_1} = \frac{M_1(1-p_1)a_1d_1}{{}_cM_1}. \tag{28}$$

In the general case, when J_1 is the ionization rate due to a combination of gamma rays, fast neutrons and slow neutrons, equation (13) can be rewritten

$$\frac{M_1(1-p_1)a_1d_1}{{}_cM_1} = (1-p_1)a_{1\gamma}D+(1-q_1)b_{1n}D+(1-r_1)c_1S \tag{29}$$

provided that the quantities a_1 and p_1 are the same for these gamma rays and those from the calibration source. This condition is satisfied with sufficient accuracy in the measurements in the experimental tanks where the average gamma ray energy was not significantly different from that of radium gamma rays (Chap. II, §15 (ii, d), p. 72). If simultaneous readings of the currents from three chambers are recorded, three equations in ${}_\gamma D$, ${}_nD$ and S each of the same form as (29) can be written down and solved. When the slow neutron flux S is small, ${}_{\gamma}D$ and ${}_{n}D$ can be found from simultaneous measurements with magnesium-argon and acetylene chambers alone, since these chambers are comparatively insensitive to slow neutrons (c_1/a_1 and c_2/a_2 are small). If the quantities associated with each of these two chambers are denoted by the suffixes 1 and 2 respectively, it can be shown that

$$ {}_{n}D = \frac{\dfrac{M_2 d_2}{{}_{c}M_2} - \dfrac{M_1 d_1}{{}_{c}M_1}}{\left(\dfrac{1-q_2}{1-p_2}\right)\dfrac{b_2}{a_2} - \left(\dfrac{1-q_1}{1-p_1}\right)\dfrac{b_1}{a_1}} \tag{30} $$

$$ {}_{\gamma}D = \frac{\dfrac{M_1 d_1}{{}_{c}M_1}\left(\dfrac{1-q_2}{1-p_2}\right)\dfrac{b_2}{a_2} - \dfrac{M_2 d_2}{{}_{c}M_2}\left(\dfrac{1-q_1}{1-p_1}\right)\dfrac{b_1}{a_1}}{\left(\dfrac{1-q_2}{1-p_2}\right)\dfrac{b_2}{a_2} - \left(\dfrac{1-q_1}{1-p_1}\right)\dfrac{b_1}{a_1}}. \tag{31} $$

When the ionization in the boron trifluoride chamber due to fast neutrons and gamma rays is negligible compared with that due to slow neutrons, the slow neutron flux is given by

$$ S = \frac{a_3 d_3}{c_3}\left(\frac{1-p_3}{1-r_3}\right)\frac{M_3}{{}_{c}M_3}. \tag{32} $$

In the general case when the ionization by fast neutrons and gamma rays is appreciable, there is an additional term involving M_1 and M_2. For this one can derive an approximate expression so that the slow neutron flux becomes

$$ S = \frac{a_3 d_3}{c_3}\left(\frac{1-p_3}{1-r_3}\right)\frac{M_3}{{}_{c}M_3} - \frac{1}{b_2 c_3}\left[\frac{M_1 d_1}{{}_{c}M_1}(b_2 a_3 - b_3 a_2) + \frac{M_2 d_2}{{}_{c}M_2} b_3 a_2\right]. \tag{33} $$

The advantage of calibrating the ionization chambers by exposure to a known dose rate is apparent from equations (30–33), namely, that currents need only be measured in arbitrary units, and the coefficients a_1, b_1, c_1 etc., enter only as ratios b_1/a_1, c_1/a_1 etc.

12. ACCURACY OF THE ESTIMATES OF DOSE RATE

(i) *Fast Neutron Dose Rate*

In the expression (30) for the fast neutron dose rate, the values of b_1/a_1 and b_2/a_2 are respectively 0·0125 and 0·770 (Tables 4, 7 and

9), and the calibrating dose rates are the same and equal to d (say) (Chap. II, §14 (iv), p. 64) so that to a good approximation one may put

$$ {}_{n}D = \frac{\left(\frac{M_2}{{}_{c}M_2} - \frac{M_1}{{}_{c}M_1}\right)d}{\frac{b_2}{a_2}\left(\frac{1-q_2}{1-p_2}\right)} \tag{34} $$

from which it follows that

$$ \frac{\delta_{n}D}{{}_{n}D} = \frac{\delta\left(\frac{M_2}{{}_{c}M_2}\right) - \delta\left(\frac{M_1}{{}_{c}M_1}\right)}{\frac{M_2}{{}_{c}M_2} - \frac{M_1}{{}_{c}M_1}} + \frac{\delta d}{d} - \frac{\delta b_2}{b_2} + \frac{\delta a_2}{a_2} - \delta\left(\frac{1-q_2}{1-p_2}\right) \tag{35} $$

where $\delta_{n}D$, δd, δb_2 ... are infinitesimal increments in ${}_{n}D$, d, b_2 ... and $(1-q_2)/(1-p_2)$ is nearly unity. These infinitesimal quantities may be regarded as representing errors of which $\delta(M_2/{}_{c}M_2)$ and $\delta(M_1/{}_{c}M_1)$ are experimental or random errors and δd, δa_2, δb_2, $\delta[(1-q_2)/(1-p_2)]$ are systematic errors. The relative values of dose rate will be effected only by the random errors. The denominator in the first term of (35) may be replaced by the approximate expression ${}_{n}Db_2/da_2$ so that the random component of error in ${}_{n}D$, i.e. the standard deviation of a single observation, is

$$ \delta_{n}D\,(\text{random}) = \frac{da_2}{b_2}\left[\left(\frac{\delta M_2}{{}_{c}M_2} - \frac{M_2 \,.\, \delta_{c}M_2}{{}_{c}M_2{}^2}\right) - \left(\frac{\delta M_1}{{}_{c}M_1} - \frac{M_1 \,.\, \delta_{c}M_1}{{}_{c}M_1{}^2}\right)\right]. \tag{36} $$

This expression includes the effect of random errors of observation together with other random errors introduced by the particular conditions of experiment, e.g. possible effects of neutron activation of the tanks and ionization chambers depending on the pattern of shutter operations, errors caused by fluctuation of pile power or disturbance of flux distribution throughout the pile. Most of these latter errors are proportional to the fast neutron dose rate which is being measured. On the other hand the purely observational error which arises, for example, from fluctuations in electrometer grid current and insulation is approximately constant, and of the order of 4 per cent of a current of 10^{-14} amp. The timing error in the Townsend balance method of ionization current measurement (Chap. II, §14 (ii), p. 61), was in all cases negligible. For the smallest currents the random errors proportional to dose are negligible, and, since M_1 and M_2 are considerably less than ${}_cM_1$ and ${}_cM_2$, we have for the observational error alone,

$$\delta_n D\,(\text{random}) = \frac{da_2}{b_2}\left(\frac{\delta M_2}{{}_cM_2} - \frac{\delta M_1}{{}_cM_1}\right). \tag{37}$$

For the acetylene and magnesium-argon pair of chambers, $d = 0{\cdot}904$ r/hr (Chap. II, §14 (iv), p. 64), $a_2/b_2 = 1{\cdot}30$ (Tables 4 and 9) and ${}_cM_1 \simeq {}_cM_2 \simeq 2{\cdot}2$ in the arbitrary units (2×10^{-12} amp) employed, and so

$$\delta_n D(\text{random}) \simeq 0{\cdot}6(\delta M_2 - \delta M_1) \tag{38}$$

δM_1 and δM_2 correspond to 2×10^{-3} in the units employed here. It follows therefore that $\delta_n D$ for low dose rates is about $0{\cdot}6\times\sqrt{2}\times2\times10^{-3}$ rads/hr, or 1·7 m rads/hr. This error which is independent of dose rate (and so of pile power) was made relatively less important by making measurements at an increased pile power. Thus, measurements of low dose rates were in fact made at ten times the standard power, and so the errors in the dose rates at the standard power were reduced by a factor of ten, i.e. to 0·17 m rads/hr.

In addition to this random error of constant order, it is assumed as explained above that there are random errors approximately proportional to the fast neutron dose rate. The magnitude of these errors can only be estimated from the internal consistency of readings at high dose rates. Thus when measuring a dose rate of 182 m rads/hr in the MAXIMUM tank (at five times the normal power) the standard deviation of the observations was 8 m rads/hr compared with the figure of 1·7 m rads/hr at low dose rates. Thus the proportional errors appear to be about 4 per cent of the dose rate being measured. Each mean value of a dose rate in Table 1 was usually derived from four individual observations, and so the standard error of the mean was calculated from $[(1{\cdot}7\times10^{-4})^2+(0{\cdot}04\ {}_nD)^2]^{\frac{1}{2}}/\sqrt{4}$ in units of rads per hour.

It is estimated that the systematic errors $\delta d/d$ and $\delta[(1-q_2)/(1-p_2)]$ are probably about 3 per cent and 2 per cent respectively. The uncertainty in the amounts of air and acetone present as impurities in the acetylene filling of the acetylene chamber might lead to errors in a_2 and b_2 of 3 per cent and 2 per cent respectively but since these errors are of the same sign the overall error in b_2/a_2 would only be 1 per cent. The only other source of systematic error in a_2 arises from a possible error in $(W/s)_{\text{air}}/(W/s)_{C_2H_2}$. This ratio is known to about 1 per cent, being dependent only upon the relative ionization currents in a given chamber when filled with air or with acetylene and exposed to radium gamma rays.

The error $\delta b_2/b_2$ is the sum of two errors, one arising from possible gross inaccuracies in the assumed shape of the energy spectrum of the fast neutrons, and the other from the lack of experimental data on the value of W for neutron recoils of various energies in acetylene. The values of bW for the acetylene chamber, given in Table 3 for the three different energy spectra, have a standard deviation of only 0·6 per cent. On the other hand the large differences between the values of W included in Table 4 suggests that the error in this quantity should be set at 10 per cent.

The sum of the individual systematic errors assigned above is 18 per cent, while the root of the sum of squares is 13 per cent. When the tissue chamber is used instead of the acetylene chamber, errors of a similar magnitude are to be expected. The errors given for the dose rates in Table 1 do not include the systematic errors.

(ii) *Gamma Ray Dose Rate*

For the discussion of errors in the gamma ray dose rates one may use the approximate expression derived from equation (31) by noting that b_1/a_1 is much less than b_2/a_2 so that

$$\frac{\delta_\gamma D}{{}_\gamma D} = \frac{\delta M_1}{M_1} - \frac{\delta_c M_1}{{}_c M_1} + \frac{\delta d}{d}. \tag{39}$$

The first and second terms represent the random errors, the former being normally much the larger. The random error in ${}_\gamma D$ is then (since $d = 0{\cdot}904$ r/hr, ${}_c M_1 = 2{\cdot}2$)

$$\delta_\gamma D = \frac{d\,.\,\delta M_1}{{}_c M_1} \simeq 0{\cdot}4\delta M_1. \tag{40}$$

It appeared from measurements at low and high dose rates as if $\delta_\gamma D$, like $\delta_n D$ above, could be regarded as made up of one part of constant order and another part approximately proportional to ${}_n D$. Thus if a measurement is made at ten times the standard power, the error in the dose rate reduced to standard power is $[(0{\cdot}8\times 10^{-4})^2 + (0{\cdot}04\ {}_n D)^2]^{\frac{1}{2}}$ and the error in the mean of four such observations is one half of this. The systematic error $\delta d/d$ associated with the dosage rate for the chamber calibration has been estimated above as 3 per cent.

(iii) *Slow Neutron Flux*

Equation (33) can be written

$$c_3 S = a_3 d_3 \left(\frac{1-p_3}{1-r_3}\right) \frac{M_3}{{}_c M_3} - b_{3n} D + a_{3\gamma} D \tag{41}$$

so that

$$\frac{\delta c_3}{c_3}S+\delta S = \frac{a_3 d_3}{c_3}\left(\frac{1-p_3}{1-r_3}\right)\frac{M_3}{{}_cM_3}$$

$$\times\left[\frac{\delta a_3}{a_3}+\frac{\delta d_3}{d_3}+\delta\left(\frac{1-p_3}{1-r_3}\right)\Big/\left(\frac{1-p_3}{1-r_3}\right)+\delta\left(\frac{M_3}{{}_cM_3}\right)\Big/\left(\frac{M_3}{{}_cM_3}\right)\right]-$$

$$-\frac{b_{3n}D}{c_3}\left(\frac{\delta b_3}{b_3}+\frac{\delta_n D}{{}_nD}\right)+\frac{a_{3\gamma}D}{c_3}\left(\frac{\delta a_3}{a_3}+\frac{\delta_\gamma D}{{}_\gamma D}\right). \qquad (42)$$

The random part of δS is the sum of the random errors

$$\frac{a_3 d_3}{c_3}\left(\frac{1-p_3}{1-r_3}\right)\delta\left(\frac{M_3}{{}_cM_3}\right),\ \frac{b_3\delta_n D}{c_3}\ \text{and}\ \frac{a_3\delta_\gamma D}{c_3}.$$

The first of these is approximately $S\delta(M_3/{}_cM_3)/(M_3/{}_cM_3)$ whilst the sum of the second and third, obtained using expressions (30) and (31), is so small (0·2 neutrons cm^{-2} sec^{-1}) that it can generally be neglected. The currents from the boron trifluoride chamber used in measuring the slow neutron flux are fairly large, so that the small observational errors are unimportant compared with the random errors due to activation and other causes (Chap. II, §12 (i), p. 53). From internal evidence the latter are about 4 per cent. Thus the whole random error in S is about 4 per cent for a single observation, or 2 per cent for the mean of four observations.

An estimate of the absolute error $\delta S/S$ could be found from equation (42) by inserting plausible values for $\delta a_3/a_3$, $\delta b_3/b_3$ ... but such a procedure is of little value because $\delta c_3/c_3$ is probably so much larger than all other errors.

The main source of error in c_3 is the energy absorption in boron trifluoride per unit flux of slow neutrons, the value of which is sensitively dependent upon the assumed energy spectrum of the neutrons. Since there is at present no information on the energy distribution of the slow neutrons in the irradiation tanks, the calculated energy absorption might well be in error by a factor of two, so the estimates of absolute flux may also be in error to the same extent. The existence of an absolute error of this magnitude in the slow neutron flux is of no practical consequence in the determination of dose rates of fast neutrons and gamma rays, since only the relative values of the ionization currents in the three chambers are required for this purpose and these are independent of the slow neutron energy spectrum (Chap. II, §4, p. 34).

13. COMPARISON OF FAST NEUTRON DOSE RATES FROM OBSERVATIONS WITH ACETYLENE, TISSUE AND ALUMINIUM-ARGON CHAMBERS

The ionization currents in the acetylene, tissue and aluminium-argon chambers (Chap. II, 14, (i), p. 58) were measured in the MAXIMUM tank with the pile operating at a steady power of 2·30 kW. Readings were taken in quick succession on the three chambers using a d.c. amplifier, type 1031. Each chamber was mounted over the centre of the floor, the tissue chamber at a height of 5·4 cm and the others at 3·5 cm. The results are recorded in Table 12 together with the radium calibrations and various correction factors.

TABLE 12

Observed ionization currents and other quantities relating to the comparison of fast neutron doses as measured with the acetylene and aluminium-argon chambers and with the tissue and aluminium-argon chambers

Chamber	Acetylene	Tissue	Al–A
Radium calibration (in arbitrary units)	4·60	5·27	8·02
Measured ionization currents (in arbitrary units) corrected to 3·5 cm above floor of MAXIMUM tank	1·41	1·78	0·55
Percentage of current caused by slow neutrons	1·1	0·3	1·6
% Saturation (at 150 V)	94·3	97·0	98·0
% Wall attenuation	2·9 (γ) 4·3 (n)	2·2 (γ) 7·2 (n)	3·0 (γ) 2·9 (n)
Coefficient a	$6{\cdot}31 \,.\, 10^8$	$5{\cdot}18 \,.\, 10^8$	$5{\cdot}11 \,.\, 10^8$
Coefficient b (variable W, modified fission spectrum)	$4{\cdot}85 \,.\, 10^8$	$4{\cdot}34 \,.\, 10^8$	†
Coefficient b (constant W, modified fission spectrum)	$5{\cdot}20 \,.\, 10^8$	$4{\cdot}62 \,.\, 10^8$	$0{\cdot}06 \,.\, 10^8$

† W is constant for all particles in argon (Chap. II, 16 (ii), p. 75)

The fast neutron and gamma ray dose rates have been calculated from the observations with the argon-filled aluminium chamber in combination with those of the acetylene chamber and also with those of the tissue chamber. It will be seen that the results given in Table 13 are consistent within the stated limits of error which were calculated by taking the root of the sums of squares of the systematic and random errors estimated above (Chap. II, §12, p. 52).

TABLE 13

Dose rates measured with the acetylene and tissue chambers, each in combination with the aluminium-argon chamber

	Acetylene and Al–A		Tissue and Al–A	
	W variable	*W* constant	*W* variable	*W* constant
Fast neutrons (m rads/hr)	276±37	267±36	288±39	270±36
Gamma rays (m r/hr)	60±12	58±12	60±12	58±12

The modified fission energy spectrum of neutrons was assumed (Chap. II, 7 (i), p. 38).

Strictly, the errors relevant to this comparison of dose rate measured by different types of chamber are somewhat less than those quoted because some of the random errors, e.g. through activation of the tank, are common to all the chambers during the short period of the measurements. For this reason, the gamma ray dose rates which are mainly affected by random errors would be expected to be well within the stated limits.

14. APPARATUS AND EXPERIMENTAL PROCEDURES

(i) *The Ionization Chambers*

The use of a small cavity ionization chamber filled with gas of different composition from the wall is not feasible for measuring neutrons of energy $\sim 10^5$ eV owing to the requirement that the dimensions of the cavity must be small compared with the ranges of the recoil particles in the gas which are $\sim$ 1 mm or less. Consideration was therefore directed at an early stage to the design of a homogeneous chamber. In order that the ionization should be a measure of the energy absorption in tissue, it was necessary that the electrodes should be constructed of a material of atomic composition as close as possible to that of tissue, particularly in its hydrogen content (Chap. II, §3 (i), p. 33).

A conducting plastic mixture of atomic composition $CH_{1 \cdot 23}$

seemed to be a suitable material for this purpose with 9·4 per cent by weight of hydrogen ('Standard Man', 10·0 per cent). It was available as pressure-moulded blocks from which the electrodes were machined, the outer electrode being fitted into an aluminium skin and the inner one fitted over an aluminium rod. A homogeneous chamber with such walls would require filling with a mixture of acetylene and ethylene and, as it appeared impracticable to provide this by continuous flow, the chamber was designed so that it could be filled and sealed off.

It was evident from the results of initial experiments with this chamber that both acetylene and ethylene were slowly taken up by the walls, with ethylene undergoing preferential absorption. The use of a gas mixture was therefore abandoned and the original lining of the chamber was replaced by another composed of polythene, polystyrene and graphite with atomic composition CH. This was filled with acetylene which flowed slowly through the chamber into the atmosphere.

In order to measure fast neutrons and gamma rays simultaneously, the acetylene chamber was used in conjunction with another which had aluminium electrodes of exactly the same size and shape. Initially the latter chamber was used with an air filling but the ^{14}N (n, p) ^{14}C reaction with slow neutrons complicated the interpretation of the measurements. Argon was selected as being a suitable substitute, its comparatively large atomic weight being a desirable factor in minimizing the ionization produced by fast neutrons.

The acetylene and argon were of commercial purity and were dried by passing over calcium chloride. The supplier stated that the acetylene had an average acetone vapour content of 3 per cent by volume and up to 1 per cent by volume of air. The combined effect of these impurities was to raise the gamma ray sensitivity by 3·4 per cent and the fast neutron sensitivity by approximately 2·4 per cent. Since the chamber was calibrated with a gamma ray source (Chap. II, §14 (iv), p. 64), the apparent neutron response was smaller than in pure acetylene by 1 per cent. The small amounts of impurities in the argon were of no consequence.

After considerably improving the accuracy of the ionization current measurements, it became apparent that there was appreciable ionization in the aluminium chamber due to protons and alpha particles resulting from fast neutron (n, p) and (n, α) reactions in the walls, in addition to that arising from beta rays from ^{28}Al formed by slow neutron capture. Accordingly most of the aluminium parts of both chambers were replaced by magnesium, this element having much smaller neutron reaction cross sections than aluminium.

A longitudinal section of the magnesium-argon chamber is shown in Fig. 7. The outer cylindrical electrode had a wall thickness of 0·45 cm, its internal diameter was 2·25 cm and its length 15 cm. The corresponding electrode of the acetylene chamber consisted of a 0·2 cm outer shell of aluminium lined with 0·2 cm of the CH plastic. The inner electrodes of both chambers were of aluminium, covered in one case with magnesium, in the other with CH plastic. The end of the amber insulator presented to the ionized gas was shielded by a magnesium 'shroud' which was fitted over the brass guard tube. This eliminated troubles due to accumulation of charges on this amber surface which resulted from the rather high electrostatic field nearby.

The diameters of these chambers were made small compared with their lengths for two reasons. Firstly, it was anticipated that the

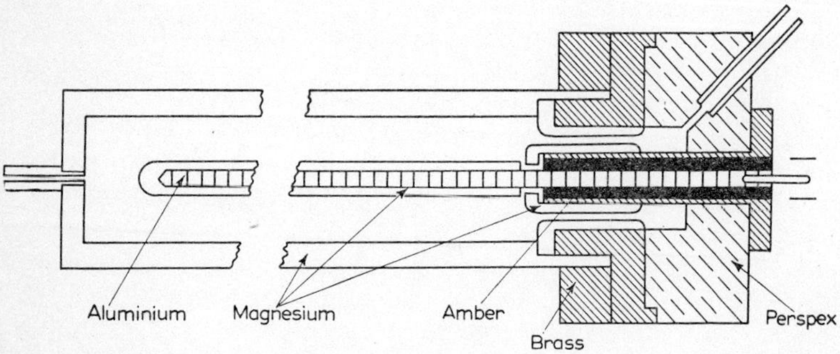

Fig. 7. Longitudinal axial section through the magnesium-argon chamber. Magnesium is shown white, brass with oblique shading, 'Perspex' with half dashed shading, aluminium with vertical shading and amber black.

radiation distribution in the tanks might show considerable gradients in two directions, so that only one dimension of the chamber could be made large, and secondly, when simultaneous measurements were made with both chambers, the errors resulting from such gradients could be minimized when the chambers were arranged alongside each other with the smallest axial separation. The amount of radiation scattered by one chamber to the other was found to be less than 1 per cent of the primary for both gamma rays and fast neutrons and has accordingly been neglected in the analysis of the observations.

Each chamber was connected to the current measuring system by a polythene insulated cable about 10 m in length which was coated with graphite and covered in the usual way. The graphite coating and outer copper braiding were connected to earth and provided adequate electrostatic shielding.

Slow neutron fluxes were measured by a boron trifluoride pulse chamber (Harwell 'teapot' type G.207/1/15) which was operated as a d.c. ionization chamber. Its electrodes were of copper 0·05 cm in thickness and were spaced 1 cm apart giving a gas volume of about 87 cc. It was filled to a pressure of 66 cm Hg at 18°C.

Most of the experimental work was carried out with the chambers described above, but a few measurements were made with a special chamber, the walls and gas filling of which had atomic compositions closely matching tissue. A rather similar chamber has been recently described by Rossi and Failla (1956). The outer electrode of our chamber consisted of a skin of 'Perspex' 0·3 cm thick which was graphited on the inside and coated with 0·1 cm of gelatin loaded with 1·28 times its weight of water and a small amount of formaldehyde to inhibit the growth of moulds. The atomic composition of the wall was computed to be $H_{1\cdot 00}\ C_{0\cdot 16}\ N_{0\cdot 04}\ O_{0\cdot 44}$. The chamber was filled with a mixture of hydrogen, oxygen, carbon dioxide and air together with water vapour at saturation pressure. Ionization measurements were made at 20°C, at which temperature the elements in the mixture could be represented by $H_{1\cdot 00}\ C_{0\cdot 15}\ N_{0\cdot 04}\ O_{0\cdot 48}$. The total pressure of the mixture was 72·3 cm Hg, the partial pressures being H_2 46 cm, H_2O 1·9 cm, CO_2 14·0 cm, O_2 7·62 cm, air 2·77 cm. Fig. 8 shows a section of the chamber. The PTFE bush provided satisfactory insulation of the collecting electrode and also formed a gas-tight seal when the taper pin was squeezed into the axial hole by turning the threaded brass end of the collecting electrode.

It was found that the gelatin lining of this chamber slowly absorbed carbon dioxide, but about 24 hours after sealing off, an approximate equilibrium gas pressure was reached. The walls were therefore saturated with this gas for 48 hours before the other components of the mixture were introduced. As a further check, the chamber was exposed to a standard 194 mg radium source immediately after filling and at regular intervals during the fast neutron measurements. These, and later tests indicated that the pressure of carbon dioxide fell at the rate of 4 per cent in 24 hours. Since the dose measurements were completed two hours after the chamber had been filled, the partial pressure of the carbon dioxide during this time can be regarded as known with sufficient precision.

(ii) *Ionization Current Measurement*

During the early stages of this work a d.c. linear amplifier (type 1031) was used for ionization current measurements, but the resistors employed in the grid circuit of the first valve were not sufficiently stable and all the later measurements were made with a different

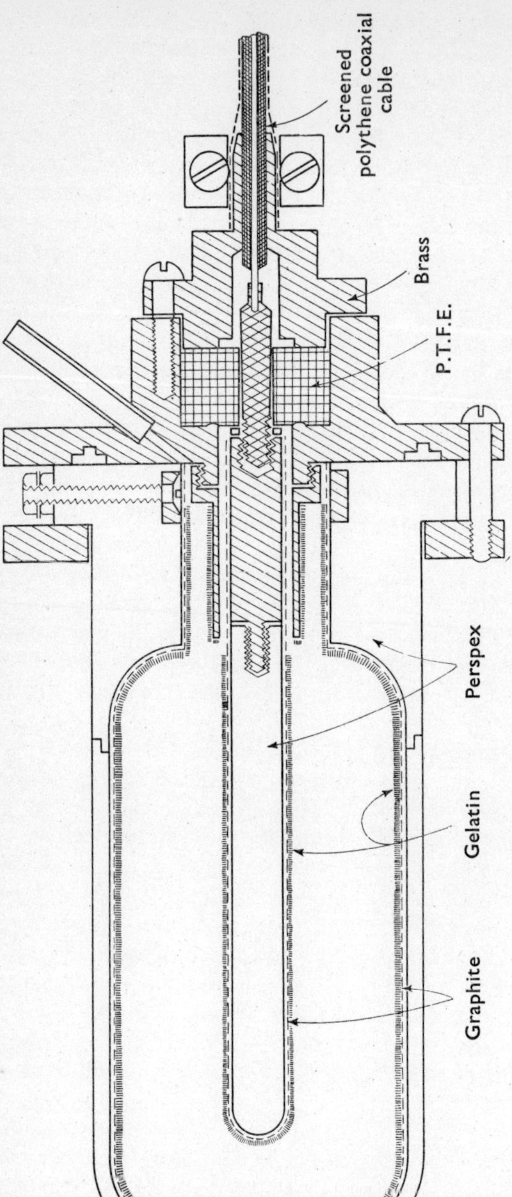

FIG. 8. Longitudinal axial section through the tissue chamber.

electrometer system by the Townsend balance method. Changes in the potential of the input terminal were detected by an FP.54 electrometer tube in a DuBridge and Brown balanced circuit. The second terminal of the condenser could be connected to 1, 2 ... or 6 standard Weston cells for final balancing, or to a potentiometer system using 2 V accumulators. In order to cover a large range of currents two alternative balance condensers were available (2·455 $\mu\mu$F and 55·09 $\mu\mu$F) and these together with the earthing switch and FP.54 tube were mounted in an evacuated chamber, thereby effectively removing parasitic ionization currents due to stray radiation.

Small drift currents of approximately 10^{-14} amp were still present a few hours after the apparatus had been switched on. Their influence on the measured ionization currents was virtually eliminated by changing the collecting field of the chamber and taking the mean of observations with the chamber voltage positive and negative. From internal evidence, it appeared that currents greater than 10^{-13} amp could be measured to an accuracy of 4 per cent or better.

For measurements in the experimental tanks with the acetylene and magnesium-argon chambers, it was customary to feed into the electrometer system the sums and differences, both positive and negative, of the two ionization currents. From a group of four such observations, errors arising from slow changes in drift currents from the amplifier and from slight drifts in power level of the pile were practically eliminated. The effect of non-uniformity of the radiation fields was overcome by taking observations with the chamber positions mutually interchanged.

(iii) *Saturation Curves*

The dependence of ionization current upon the collecting voltage was investigated with the acetylene and magnesium chambers filled with hydrogen, acetylene, oxygen, carbon dioxide and argon, and also with these gases nearly saturated with water vapour at 20°C. Measurements were also made with the tissue chamber filled with its special gas mixture.

The chambers were exposed in the MAXIMUM tank with the pile operating at 3 kW, at which power the dose rates were 364 m rads/hr of fast neutrons and 69·5 mr/hr of gamma rays, and also in some cases to radium gamma rays at 5 r/hr. The saturation curves in some typical cases are shown in Fig. 9 where the ionization current, represented as a fraction of the extrapolated saturation current, is plotted against the minimum field in the chamber, $V/b \ln(b/a)$ volts/cm, where $V =$ chamber volts, a and b are the radii of the inner and outer electrodes. The minimum field, which was approximately one fifth of the maximum field in all cases, is probably the most relevant parameter for the acetylene and tissue chambers, since a large fraction of the ionization in these cases occurs near the outer electrode.

From the results it was found that for fast neutrons the corrections to be applied to the current measurements at the usual collecting voltages of 360 were respectively 3·2 per cent and 2·7 per cent for acetylene and magnesium chambers with their normal

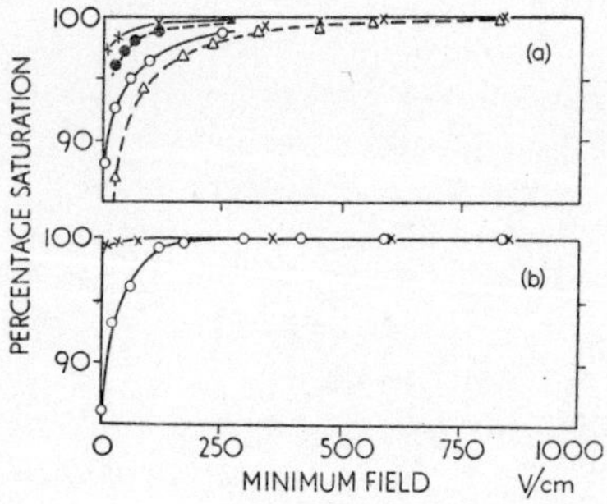

FIG. 9. Saturation curves for chambers with various gas fillings.
(a) CH chamber with H_2 —x— O_2 --●--, A —o—, C_2H_2 --Δ--;
(b) Mg chamber with H_2 —x—, A —o—

gas fillings. Under the same conditions the corrections for the gamma ray component were negligibly small.

For each of the gases investigated the collecting field for a given degree of saturation was approximately inversely proportional to the mobility of the positive ions. The presence of water vapour at a pressure of 2 cm Hg did not significantly affect the saturation curve for any gas.

(iv) *Calibration of the Chambers*

The calibration of the ionization chambers was carried out at regular intervals by exposure to a standard radium source thereby providing a rapid check on both the radiation sensitivity of the chamber and the performance of the current measuring apparatus. The routine tests were carried out at 2 hourly intervals during a long run of observations. The radium source of 194·0 mg in a platinum container of 0·5 mm wall was mounted on a light 'Perspex' frame which could be attached to the chamber by two spring loaded 'V' clamps. This arrangement ensured very precise location of the source with respect to the chamber, the actual distance from source to centre of chamber being 18·4 cm. It was not suitable, however, for absolute calibrations owing to considerable non-uniformity of the radiation flux within the chamber due to the close proximity of the source.

Absolute calibrations were carried out in the following way. The chamber and the radium source, mounted in the equatorial plane of the chamber on a thin aluminium rod, were isolated as far as practicable from surrounding scattering objects. The distance between the chamber and source was defined by a 40 cm spacer placed between them. After correcting for radium salt absorption, the average dose rate at the fast neutron and gamma chambers was found by calculation to be 0·904 r/hr, assuming 8·4 r/hr at 1 cm from a 1 mg point source. The corresponding figures for the boron trifluoride and tissue chambers were 0·907 r/hr and 0·859 r/hr.

15. ENERGY OF GAMMA RAYS IN THE IRRADIATION TANKS

In the majority of fast neutron measurements carried out in the course of this work, the ionization in the acetylene and magnesium-argon chambers due to the gamma ray component of the radiation field was at least of the same order of magnitude as that due to fast neutrons. It was therefore essential to estimate the ionization due to the gamma component as accurately as possible. Since the relative gamma sensitivities of the chambers (coefficient a of Table 9) are slightly dependent upon the radiation energy (Chap. II, §9, p. 47), it was necessary to investigate the energy of the gamma rays experimentally. Two methods were used.

(1) The 'attenuation' method, in which the ionization was measured as a function of the thickness of an absorbing sheath which enclosed the chamber. For a thin sheath it can be shown to a first approximation, that the ionization is reduced by a factor $\exp\{-mnZ(\sigma_a+\tau+\kappa)\}$ where n is the number of atoms of atomic number Z per unit mass, σ_a and τ are defined in Chap. II, §5, p. 36, κ is the cross section per electron for pair production and m the mass per unit area of the wall. From the values of σ_a, τ and κ given by Davisson and Evans (1952) one can find the energy of the homogeneous gamma rays which have the same attenuation coefficient as that observed with the unknown radiation.

(2) The 'emission' method, in which the ionization was measured in a number of chambers with walls of widely different atomic numbers. In this method all the chambers had the same gas filling (argon), and were exposed to the same radiation field, and so the ionization per unit mass of gas in a cavity with walls composed of atoms of type i was proportional to $(\sigma_a+\tau+\kappa)_i/s_i$, by equation 12, where $E = Gn_iZ_i(\sigma_a+\tau+\kappa)_i$ and s_i is the electronic stopping

power of the wall for secondary electrons. The ratios of the currents in different chambers in conjunction with data on $(\sigma_a+\tau+\kappa)$ and s yielded the energy of the equivalent homogeneous gamma radiation.

(i) *Experimental Details*

In order to minimize the ionization by fast neutrons, it was necessary to select for the chamber walls elements with small neutron cross sections. For the purpose of these measurements the outer electrode of the acetylene chamber was replaced by graphite (2·5 mm), zirconium (0·6 mm) or lead (0·21 mm) and the inner electrode covered with similar material of the same thickness. Argon was used throughout as a gas filling.

All measurements in the irradiation tanks were made with the chamber axes horizontal 4 cm above the centre of the floor. No observations were attempted in the MAXIMUM tank in view of the very large neutron flux, nor in the GAMMA tank because of the low radiation intensity.

Ionization currents were measured when the chambers were exposed to the 194·0 mg radium source and to a ^{60}Co source of comparable strength, using the same geometry as that employed in the chamber calibrations (Chap. II, §14 (iv), p. 64). The purpose of these observations was to provide a check on the methods of energy measurement and to give information on the relative volumes of the chambers. The latter was required in order to correlate the data for the different chambers using the emission method.

For the attenuation experiments, absorbing sheaths of aluminium and lead of various thicknesses were made to fit closely around the outer electrodes.

(ii) *Results*

(a) *Attenuation Method*

The results of the attenuation measurements are summarized in Table 14.

Observations were carried out in the MEDIUM and MINIMUM tanks with the shutters open and closed (indicated in the table by (O) and (C) respectively). In all cases the thickness of the absorber was sufficiently small to produce less than 10 per cent attenuation. The value of the observed attenuation coefficient in column (3) was obtained by plotting the logarithm of the ionization current against absorber thickness and judging by eye the best fitting straight line. The energies of homogeneous gamma rays which would suffer the same attenuation, according to Davisson and Evans (1952) are given in column (4). These energies are only very approximate since the effective thickness of a cylindrical attenuator is appreciably greater

TABLE 14

The energies of gamma rays in the irradiation tanks and of radium and ^{60}Co as found from measurements of their attenuation

Radn. source	Chamber wall (1)	Ab-sorber (2)	Obs. attn. coeff. (cm^{-1}) (3)	Equiv. gamma energy (MeV) (4)	Attn. corr. factor (5)	Corrected attn. coeff. (cm^{-1}) (6)	Gamma ray energy (MeV) (7)
MED (O)	Mg	Pb	2·6	0·36	1·30	2·0	0·40
MED (O)	Pb	Pb	1·0	0·56	1·70	0·59	0·80
MED (C)	Pb	Pb	3·1	0·33	1·70	1·8	0·42
MIN (O)	C	Pb	1·3	0·49	1·29	1·0	0·56
MIN (O)	Mg	Pb	0·9	0·60	1·29	0·70	0·70
MIN (C)	C	Pb	2·1	0·39	1·29	1·6	0·42
MIN (C)	Mg	Pb	1·2	0·50	1·29	0·93	0·58
MED (O)	Mg	Al	0·15	0·07	1·29	0·12	0·09
MED (O)	Mg	Al	0·20	0·06	1·29	0·16	0·08
MIN (C)	Mg	Al	0·19	0·06	1·29	0·15	0·07
Radium	C	Al	0·074	0·9	1·30	0·057	~ 2
Radium	C	Pb	0·7	0·70	1·29	0·54	0·86
Radium	Pb	Pb	1·9	0·41	1·67	1·14	0·52
^{60}Cobalt	C	Pb	0·5	0·91	1·29	0·39	1·22
^{60}Cobalt	Pb	Pb	0·7	0·70	1·67	0·42	1·10

Note. (O) denotes tank shutter open
(C) denotes tank shutter closed

than the thickness measured normal to its surface. A quantitative estimate of the correction factor is clearly required.

Considering first the primary radiation which lies in a plane at right angles to the chamber axis, the appropriate correction factors have been calculated on two different assumptions:

(i) that the tracks of secondary electrons originating in a small element of the wall are distributed isotropically in laboratory coordinates, and

(ii) that the secondary electrons are emitted only in the same direction as the incident radiation.

The attenuation coefficients are found to be larger than those for normal incidence through a plane sheet by factors which are respectively

$$\frac{E(\alpha)-\sin\alpha}{\frac{\pi}{2}(1-\sin\alpha)} \tag{43}$$

and

$$\frac{4}{3\pi(1-\sin\alpha)}\{(1+\operatorname{cosec}^2\alpha)E(\alpha)+(1-\operatorname{cosec}^2\alpha)K(\alpha)-2\sin\alpha\} \tag{44}$$

where $\sin \alpha = a/b$, a = int. radius of outer electrode, b = ext. radius of outer electrode and $E(\alpha)$ and $K(\alpha)$ are the complete elliptic integrals tabulated by Jahnke and Emde (1945). These factors are shown graphically in Fig. 10 as functions of $\sin \alpha$.

As the actual distribution in space of the secondary electron tracks is intermediate between the assumed distributions (i) and (ii) but is

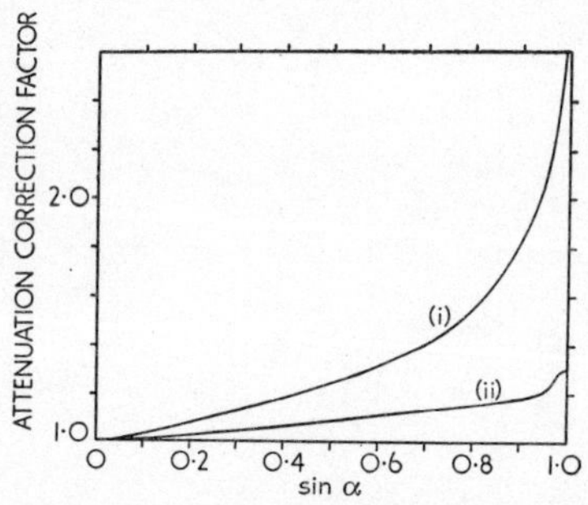

FIG. 10. The correction factor for wall attenuation in a cylindrical chamber; (i) secondary particles emitted isotropically (expression 43), (ii) ditto in the forward direction only (expression 44), where $\sin \alpha$ = (internal radius of chamber) ÷ (external radius).

otherwise not amenable to simple treatment, it was decided to adopt the average of the two factors (43) and (44). In most cases the differences between them were quite small (cf. Table 10).

When the chamber wall and the absorbing sheath have different compositions, the problem is more complex. An approximate treatment indicates that the attenuation factor in such cases is close to that which would apply to a wall composed of a uniform mixture of the sheath and wall with the corresponding proportions and the same overall thickness. For simplicity it has been assumed that the attenuation with dissimilar layers is equal to that of the uniform 'mixture'.

Since each chamber was exposed to gamma rays coming from all directions beneath it, one should make allowance for the additional attenuation of radiation not in the plane at right angles to its axis. No information on the angular distribution of the gamma radiation in the tanks was available, but the considerable attenuation in the floor by the 2-in. layer of lead ($\sim e^{-3}$) suggested that the primary gamma ray energy flux per unit solid angle would decrease fairly rapidly with increasing deviation from the vertical. For a radiation distribution with azimuthal symmetry, the average value of the cosine of the angle between the chamber axis and a beam at an angle ϕ from the vertical is $(2 \sin \phi)/\pi$, so that even if ϕ is 30°, the effective wall thickness will only be increased by the factor sec 18·5°, i.e., by 1·05. It seems likely therefore, that the additional attenuation of radiation oblique to the chamber axis will not seriously influence the ionization and that the errors introduced by neglecting it will be smaller than the errors in the observed coefficients.

The correction factors for the attenuation coefficient calculated as described above are given in column (5) of Table 14. When the attenuation coefficients in column (3) are divided by the correction factors in column (5) obtained from (43) and (44), one finds the coefficients given in column (6). The equivalent gamma ray energies appear in column (7).

Using lead absorbers the energies found for ^{60}Co are very close to the true values, whilst those for radium correspond to the more readily absorbed components of lower energy. It will be noticed that the observations with aluminium absorbers yield very different gamma ray energies from those obtained with lead. The most important source of error in the interpretation of the data for aluminium is probably the fact that the chamber and its sheath are regarded as 'thin' even when their combined thickness is between 4 and 10 mm. Thus the correct absorption coefficient should be intermediate between $(\sigma_a+\tau+\kappa)$ and $(\sigma_a+\sigma_s+\tau+\kappa)$. For gamma rays of 0·5 MeV the ratio $(\sigma_a+\sigma_s+\tau+\kappa)/(\sigma_a+\tau+\kappa)$ is 1·22 for lead and 3·2 for aluminium. Thus, the apparent attenuation coefficient in aluminium would be expected to depend more critically on the effect of wall scattering in a thick wall, than in the case of lead. This source of uncertainty, coupled with the fact that $(\sigma_a+\tau+\kappa)$ changes by only 10 per cent from 0·3 MeV to 1·2 MeV, suggests that the results for aluminium should be given very little weight compared with those for lead. The average of the results with lead attenuation for the energy of the gamma rays in the tanks was $0{\cdot}56\pm0{\cdot}14$ MeV.

(b) *Emission Method*

The relative volumes of the chambers were first deduced by exposing them to a source of ^{60}Co under conditions of identical geometry. The results are given in Table 15.

The wall attenuation factors listed in column (2) were calculated by the method described above (assuming an energy of 1·2 MeV). The energy distribution of the secondary electrons at the inner surface of a chamber wall was found by the method of Cormack and Johns (1952). From the stopping power tables of Aron, Hoffmann and Williams (1949) the ionization due to electrons in each of the energy ranges 0–0·1 MeV, 0·1–0·2 MeV, ... was calculated and, by summation, the mean effective value of stopping power for the whole

TABLE 15

Derivation of the relative volumes of chambers used in estimation of gamma ray energies by the 'emission' method

Chamber wall	Observed ionization current (arbitrary units) (1)	Calc. wall atten. factor (2)	Corrected ionization current rel. to Mg (3)	$\frac{s_{Mg}}{s_i}$ (4)	$\frac{(\sigma_a+\tau+\kappa)M_i}{(\sigma_a+\tau+\kappa)_{Mg}}$ (5)	$\frac{V_i}{V_{Mg}}$ (6)
C	1·646	1·032	0·860	0·91	0·999	0·95
Mg	1·925	1·027	(1·00)	(1·00)	(1·000)	(1·00)
Zr	5·47	1·017	2·81	1·26	1·055	2·12
Pb	6·45	1·065	3·47	1·46	1·625	1·47

energy distribution. These stopping power ratios are given in column (4) of Table 15. When the ionization currents (corrected for wall attenuation) were divided by

$$\frac{s_{Mg}}{s_i} \cdot \frac{(\sigma_a+\tau+\kappa)_i}{(\sigma_a+\tau+\kappa)_{Mg}}$$

the relative gas volumes given in the last column were found.

The ionization currents in chambers with graphite, magnesium, zirconium and lead walls, exposed in the MEDIUM and MINIMUM tanks, were measured with shutters and shields in the open and closed positions. Knowing the relative gas volumes of the chambers one can find the relative ionization currents per unit mass and these are given in Table 16, corrected for wall attenuation. From each of them a value of the energy of the equivalent homogeneous gamma radiation has been found in the following way. The quantity $(\sigma_a+\tau+\kappa)$ which is proportional to the ionization current per unit mass of gas, has been calculated for each chamber for a number of gamma ray energies on the simplifying assumption that the average energy of the secondary electrons is one-fifth of the energy of the photon, this being the average value of the fraction found in the calculations of effective stopping power described above for ^{60}Co gamma radiation. Since the relative electronic stopping powers change rather slowly with energy around 1 MeV, this approximation is sufficiently accurate. The relative values of $(\sigma_a+\tau+\kappa)$ were plotted as functions of photon energy and from this curve the energy of the homogeneous gamma radiation corresponding to each of the observed ionization currents was found. The results are given in the lower half of Table 16.

TABLE 16

Energies of gamma rays in the irradiation tanks as found by the 'emission' method

	Radiation source	Chamber	Shutter open		Shutter closed	
			Shield open	Shield closed	Shield open	Shield closed
Ionization currents per unit mass of gas relative to magnesium	MED tank	Zr Pb	1·43 3·95	1·44 —	1·48 5·23	— —
	MIN tank	C Zr	0·90 1·48	0·88 1·47	0·90 1·54	0·86 1·36
Effective gamma ray energies (MeV)	MED tank	Zr/Mg Pb/Mg Pb/Zr	0·88 0·78 0·75	0·84 — —	0·78 0·65 0·62	— — —
	MIN tank	Zr/Mg Zr/C	0·78 0·74	0·79 0·72	0·70 0·70	1·05 0·83
Mean energy (MeV)			0·79±0·05		0·76±0·13	

The ratio of currents in the magnesium and carbon chambers is of no value for the determination of energy in this region, since $(\sigma_a+\tau+\kappa)_{Mg}/(\sigma_a+\tau+\kappa)_C$, is very nearly constant (Chap. II, §5, p. 36).

The results do not suggest any marked influence of the positions of either shields or shutters on the effective energy, the mean value of which is 0·78±0·10 MeV. As a check on this method of estimation of gamma-ray energies, ionization current measurements were made in carbon, magnesium, zirconium and lead chambers exposed to a radium source. The currents per unit mass of argon had the relative magnitudes 0·894, 1·00, 1·554, and 4·08. Following the above method it was deduced that the equivalent gamma ray energies were 0·70 MeV (Zr/Mg), 0·67 MeV (Zr/C), 0·76 MeV (Pb/Mg), 0·75 MeV (Pb/C), and 0·78 MeV (Pb/Zr). The energy of 0·76 from the Pb/Mg ratio may be compared with the value derived from the gamma ray spectrum of Ra (B+*C*) given by Ellis and Aston (1930), allowance being made for absorption in the 0·5 mm platinum filter of the source. Each line was given a weight proportional to its energy, excitation, and absorption coefficient $(\sigma_a+\tau+\kappa)$. The ratio of the summation for lead and magnesium corresponded to an effective energy of 0·78 MeV, in satisfactory agreement with the experimental figure above.

(c) *The Means of the Results by Both Methods*

In this part of the experiment, the ionization current measurements in the irradiation tanks had a rather low accuracy owing to the limitations of the d.c. amplifier used (Chap. II, §14 (ii), p. 61). The results do not show good internal consistency, particularly those for the attenuation method. Some of the inconsistencies may have been due to neutron activation effects for which no correction was made.

If the values of equivalent energy of the tank radiation obtained by methods (1) and (2) viz $0{\cdot}56 \pm 0{\cdot}14$ MeV and $0{\cdot}78 \pm 0{\cdot}12$ MeV are given weights inversely proportional to their standard deviations one finds a mean value of $0{\cdot}68 \pm 0{\cdot}08$ Mev. The average of the seven values for radium gamma rays, is $0{\cdot}73 \pm 0{\cdot}04$ MeV.

(d) *Conclusion*

From the experimental investigations described above one may conclude that the average energy of the gamma radiation in the experimental tanks is close to that of radium gamma rays. Gray's (1936) experimental values of the relative stopping powers of light elements for the secondary electrons from radium gamma rays can therefore be used for the gamma radiation in the experimental tanks.

16. ENERGY LOSS PER ION PAIR IN GASES

If the number of ions produced by each fast recoil particle in an ionization chamber were strictly proportional to its energy loss in the gas, the observed ionization in a homogeneous chamber would be proportional to the energy absorbed in the gas. On the other hand, if the average energy lost by a particle in creating a pair of ions, W, depended upon its speed and mass, the form of dependence and the initial energies of the recoil particles would have to be known before the total ionization and total energy absorbed in the gas could be related. The published experimental data on W for electrons, protons and alpha particles are still very incomplete, whilst none are available for the heavier neutron recoils in tissue-like materials. In the following review an attempt has been made to integrate these data in order to deduce the best values of W for each type of secondary ionizing particle produced in our chambers.

Observations by Gerbes (1935) on the energy per ion pair for fast electrons in air, together with those of Eisl (see Gerbes, 1935) and Pigge (1934) were found by Gerbes to fit the empirical expression

$$W_e(\epsilon) = 31{\cdot}6 + 5{\cdot}27(\epsilon - I)^{-1/2} \pm 0{\cdot}08 \text{ e}V/\text{ion pair} \qquad (45)$$

where ϵ is the initial energy of the electron in keV and I the ionization potential of air (= $1{\cdot}7 \,.\, 10^{-2}$ keV). The range of electron energies covered by the experimental data was 0·3 to 60 keV. By contrast, Freund (1935) and Breunig (1936) using an experimental method quite different from that of Eisl and Gerbes, concluded that W was almost constant at 32 ± 2 eV for electrons in air in the range 75 eV to 300 eV. Gerbes (1937) found that for electrons in oxygen, nitrogen carbon dioxide and argon, W showed a variation with energy very closely similar to that in air in the energy range 10 to 40 keV.

The experimental data for protons and alpha particles in various gases published before 1944, have been critically reviewed by Gray (1944). He concluded that for alpha particles in hydrogen, helium, neon and argon, the energy per ion pair W_α was sensibly constant in the energy range 0·33 to 3·4 MeV. With air W_α appeared to increase steadily as the energy of the particle diminished, the rate of increase being about one half of that shown by electrons of the same speed (equation (45)). For protons in air, Gray found that the evidence pointed to a value of W 4 per cent greater than that of an alpha particle of the same speed.

The expression (45) is open to criticism on the ground that the instantaneous rate of energy dissipation per ion pair $^*W_e$ which is derived from (45) tends to zero as the instantaneous value of the electron energy $^*\epsilon$ tends to I. This fact was apparently not realized by Gerbes, owing to an error in his derivation of $^*W_e$ from W_e. For $(^*\epsilon - I)$ small, (45) yields

$$^*W_e(^*\epsilon) = \frac{10{\cdot}54(^*\epsilon - I)}{^*\epsilon} \tag{46}$$

which tends to zero as $^*\epsilon - I$ tends to zero whereas physically $^*W_e$ must tend to infinity.

The accuracy of the experimental points on which (45) is based is such that they would fit just as closely other expressions of different form. Since theoretical considerations have so far given no indication of the likely dependence of $^*W_e$ upon $^*\epsilon$ apart from the prediction that it should become approximately constant at high energies (Fano, 1946), the authors have assumed an expression which is effectively equivalent to that of Gerbes at high energies, viz.

$$\frac{^*W_e(^*\epsilon)}{W_e(\infty)} = 1 + \lambda(^*\epsilon - I)^{-1/2} \tag{47}$$

where λ and $W_e(\infty)$ (the value of $^*W_e$ as $^*\epsilon$ tends to ∞) are numerical constants whose values are adjusted to give the best fit with the experimental points. The number of ions produced by an electron of initial energy ϵ when it is stopped in air is $\epsilon/W_e(\epsilon)$, which for convenience can be written as

$$\frac{\epsilon}{W_e(\infty)} \cdot \frac{W_e(\infty)}{W_e(\epsilon)}$$

where the quantity $W_e(\infty)/W_e(\epsilon)$ is the ionization efficiency of the electron (relative to one of 'infinite' energy). From (47) it can be shown that $W_e(\infty)/W_e(\epsilon)$ is given by

$$\frac{W_e(\infty)}{W_e(\epsilon)} = \frac{1}{\epsilon}\left\{(\epsilon-I)-2\lambda(\epsilon-I)^{\frac{1}{2}}+2\lambda^2\ln\left[1+\frac{(\epsilon-I)^{1/2}}{\lambda}\right]\right\}. \tag{48}$$

When $(\epsilon - I)$ is small

$$\frac{W_e(\infty)}{W_e(\epsilon)} \simeq \frac{2(\epsilon-I)^{3/2}}{3\lambda\epsilon} \tag{49}$$

and when ϵ is large

$$\frac{W_e(\infty)}{W_e(\epsilon)} \simeq \frac{1}{1+2\lambda\epsilon^{-1/2}} \tag{50}$$

Since the cross sections for excitation and ionization of gas molecules by a charged particle are primarily dependent upon the speed of the particle, an expression of the same form as (47) would be expected to hold for a heavy charged particle. For particle energies much larger than the ionization potential, $(\epsilon-I)$ can be replaced by ϵ and equations (47) and (48) can be written in the more general form

$$\frac{{}^*W({}^*v)}{W(\infty)} = 1+\mu\frac{v_0}{{}^*v} \tag{51}$$

$$\frac{W(\infty)}{W(v)} = 1-2\mu\frac{v_0}{v}+2\mu^2\frac{v_0^2}{v^2}\ln\left(1+\frac{v}{\mu v_0}\right) \tag{52}$$

where $\mu v_0=\lambda\sqrt{(2/M)}$, M being the mass of the particle, v its initial speed and v_0 ($\equiv e^2/\hbar = 2{\cdot}188 \,.\, 10^8$ cm/sec) the speed of the electron in the first Bohr orbit of the hydrogen atom. If the ionization efficiency were a function of particle speed only, then for all particles μ would have a unique value. For most gases, it has been found that $\mu \sim 1/\pi$ so the term $\mu\,(v_0/{}^*v) \sim t/t_0$ where t is the time of passage of the charged particle across the molecule and t_0 the time of revolution of the valence electrons. Thus the physical interpretation of (51) is that the ionization efficiency is approximately unity when $t \ll t_0$ and does not decrease appreciably until $t \sim t_0$.

(i) *Experimental Work since 1944*

Since 1944, a considerable amount of experimental work has been published on the values of W for ionizing particles, mainly alphas, in several gases. The methods principally employed were:

(1) Measurement of the number of ions resulting from the total absorption within the ionization chamber of a single particle or a pair of particles, e.g. those from $^{10}B(n, \alpha)\,^{7}Li$, using

- (*a*) a fast counter with electron collection, e.g. a pulse ionization chamber or proportional counter and a fast linear amplifier feeding a pulse analyzer,
- (*b*) a recording electrometer system which has a very much longer time constant than (*a*) due to the inertia of the moving parts.

(2) Measurement of the steady current in an ionization chamber due to particles which are completely stopped in the gas and which enter the chamber at a rate determined independently.

Probably the most important single source of error common to all experimental methods is failure to collect all the ions produced. Recombination losses can be kept small by using low gas pressures and adequate collecting fields, the latter preferably at right angles to the tracks of the ionizing particles. These conditions appear to have been met by Jesse, Forstat and Sadauskis (1950) and by Jesse and Sadauskis (1950, 1952, 1953, 1955) in their experiments with alpha particles. These workers followed the somewhat unusual practice of measuring ionization pulses due to single particles by an electrometer feeding a pen recorder. The collection times could therefore be very long ($\sim$ 1 sec) compared with those which are possible using conventional fast pulse measuring techniques ($\sim$ few μsec).

(ii) *Energy per Ion Pair in Argon*

Most of the results obtained with fast counters filled with argon (Cranshaw and Harvey, 1948; Rhodes, Franzen and Stephens, 1950; Tunnicliffe and Ward, 1952) are consistent with the hypothesis that in this gas the value of W for alpha particles and other heavy ionizing particles increases with diminishing particle speed. However, this interpretation of the experimental data now appears open to doubt. In the first place Jesse and Sadauskis (1952) have shown that for alpha particles in the inert gases W is particularly susceptible to errors arising from small traces of impurity, so that an apparent dependence of W upon particle speed might well arise from the presence of a small percentage of foreign gas which is added to argon in pulse chambers. Hanna (1950) has also pointed out that secondary photoelectrons from the electrodes arising from argon atoms in excited metastable states might be missed in fast counters. Since the cross section for excitation increases relative to that for ionization as the particle energy diminishes, failure to collect such electrons could lead to an apparent increase in W. Finally De Juren and Rosenwasser (1954) have recently found evidence of columnar recombination along the tracks of the particles from the reaction $^{10}B(n, \alpha)^{7}Li$ in pulse ionization chambers filled with argon and a small percentage of carbon dioxide or methane. Such recombination losses would be relatively large for slow ionizing particles and would cause a progressive increase in W with diminishing particle speed.

Recently, Jesse and Sadauskis (1955) have extended an earlier investigation (1950) and have found strong evidence in support of the conclusion of Gray (1944) that for the inert gases and hydrogen W_{α} is probably independent of particle energy. The case of alpha particles in helium has been examined theoretically by Erskine (1954), who finds that W_{α} is substantially constant between 1 MeV and 6 MeV at 41 eV/ion pair, a value which agrees well with recent measurements in very pure helium (Bortner and Hurst, 1953; Jesse and Sadauskis 1952).

There is excellent agreement amongst most of the recent determinations of the energy per ion pair in argon for alpha particles from ^{210}Po(5·3 MeV). Haeberli, Huber and Baldinger (1953) found 26·3 eV, whilst Jesse and Sadauskis (1953) and Bortner and Hurst (1953) both found 26·4 eV. Sharpe (1952) using ^{239}Pu alpha particles (5·16 MeV) reported the value of 26·3 eV.

Absolute values of W for electrons in argon have been reported by Nicodemus (1946) and Valentine (1952). For electrons from tritium ($\bar{\epsilon} \approx 6$ keV), Nicodemus found 26·9 eV/ion pair, whilst Valentine, using electrons from ^{37}A ($\bar{\epsilon} \approx 3$ keV) found 27·0 eV/ion pair. Valentine (1952) and Valentine and Curran (1952) concluded that the value of W for electrons was identical—within the limits of experimental error—to that for polonium alpha particles for which they found 25·9 eV/ion pair. In this work Valentine and Curran employed slow collection in their measurements of ionization currents, but it should be noted that the argon used was not pure. Jesse and Sadauskis (1955) have observed the relative ionization currents due to alpha particles and to electrons from tritium and ^{63}Ni ($\bar{\epsilon} \approx 15$ keV) and have concluded that W_{α}/W_{e} is independent of the energies of the electron and alpha particle in the inert gases and hydrogen.

The importance of observations in argon arises from the fact that the values of W in other gases have usually been measured relative to argon. Although the earlier work with fast counters appeared to indicate that W in argon increased with diminishing particle energy, it now seems to the writers that the weight of evidence is in favour of a constant value for alpha particles, electrons and other ionizing particles in argon and similarly for the other inert gases and hydrogen. Such an assumption has therefore been made in interpreting the results for acetylene and other gases.

(iii) *Energy per Ion Pair in Acetylene*

Jesse and Sadauskis (1955) have measured the total number of ions produced by a single alpha particle from ^{210}Po when it is stopped in acetylene and in other hydrocarbon gases. They have also found the relative ionization yields from alpha particles which were slowed down to about 1·2 MeV before they entered the chamber, and from electrons from tritium and ^{63}Ni. Their results are given in columns (2), (3), (6) and (7) of Table 17, those for electrons being derived on the assumption that the absolute value of W for electrons in argon is equal to that for alpha particles, viz. 26·35 eV.

If the value of W_α in each of these gases were a function of particle speed of the type given by equation (52), one could find the quantities μ and $W_\alpha(\infty)$ from the observed ratios $W_\alpha(1{\cdot}2\text{ MeV})/W_\alpha(5{\cdot}3\text{ MeV})$. Although such a procedure is open to criticism, it has been carried out with the results shown in columns (4) and (5). It is evident that $W_\alpha(\infty)$ is in all cases close to W_e, the average value of the ratio $W_e/W_\alpha(\infty)$ for all gases being $0{\cdot}997 \pm 0{\cdot}003$. The average energy of electrons from ^{63}Ni and ^{3}H is 10 keV which corresponds to a speed of $26{\cdot}4\,v_0$. For an alpha particle of this speed, one finds from equation (52) that $W_\alpha/W_\alpha(\infty)$ is 1·017, taking $\mu = 0{\cdot}25$, the average of the values in column (4) of Table 17.

TABLE 17

Energy per ion pair (eV) for hydrocarbon gases
(from Jesse and Sadauskis, 1955)

(1) Gas	(2) W_α(1·2 MeV)	(3) W_α(5·3 MeV)	(4) μ	(5) $W_\alpha(\infty)$	(6) $W_e(^3H)$	(7) $W_e(^{63}Ni)$
C_2H_2	29·0	27·5	0·21	26·1	26·1	—
C_2H_4	29·8	28·0	0·26	26·2	—	26·3
C_2H_6	28·5	26·6	0·28	24·8	24·9	24·6
CH_4	31·0	29·2	0·25	27·5	27·3	—

Comparison of the ratio 1·017 with the value 0·997 derived above suggests that the value of μ is smaller for electrons than for alpha particles in the hydrocarbon gases.

Apart from the recent work of Jesse and Sadauskis (1955) discussed above, there are no other data bearing directly upon the dependence of W upon particle velocity in acetylene. Some measurements of the ionization by ThC and ThC′ recoils from alpha disintegrations have, however, been made in methane by Stone and Cochran (1954). The values of W were found to be 137 eV/ion pair and 120 eV/ion pair respectively, which correspond to 5·00 and 4·38 times $W_\alpha(\infty)$. The initial energies of these particles are 0·118 and 0·170 MeV and if their ionization efficiencies conform to relation (52) then the values of μ are 0·41 and 0·40 respectively.

The absolute value of W for alpha particles from ^{210}Po in acetylene is given by Jesse and Sadauskis (1953) as 27·5 eV/ion. Dainty (1950) measured the relative values for acetylene and air using ^{239}Pu alpha particles and found precisely the same ratio as Jesse and Sadauskis. No absolute values for electrons have been published and the only relative values, apart from data of Jesse and Sadauskis (1955) discussed above, are those found by Failla and Rossi (1954) and by Munson (unpublished). With electrons from ^{35}S, Failla and Rossi found that the energy per ion pair in acetylene was 0·780 times that in air, whilst Munson, from measurements of the ionization due to secondary electrons from radium (average energy $\sim$ 300 keV), found the ratio 0·76. Both results are in fair agreement with the figure 0·766 from the work of Jesse and Sadauskis (1955).

From the above analysis it appears that equation (52) does provide a consistent description of the experimental results, the values of μ for electrons, alpha particles and heavy recoils in methane showing a relatively small progressive change with particle mass. A small change is not surprising since the ionization efficiency depends upon the relative cross sections for ionization, excitation and other modes of energy loss and the latter will not depend simply upon particle speed.

(iv) *Energy per Ion Pair in Nitrogen, Oxygen, Air, Carbon Dioxide, Water Vapour and Boron Trifluoride*

Recently published values of energy per ion pair, relative to argon, in each of the gases used in the tissue chamber and in boron trifluoride are shown in Table 18. In three cases measurements were not made in argon, whilst in another it seemed likely that the result for argon was 3 per cent low, due to an error in the assumed electronic stopping power for argon. The relative values of W in these cases are normalized by reference to the average values for air.

TABLE 18

Energy per ion pair (relative to argon, $W_A = 26{\cdot}35$ eV) for boron trifluoride and the gases in the tissue chamber

Reference	Particle	Initial energy	Values of W(gas)/W(argon) A	H_2	N_2	O_2	air	CO_2	H_2O	BF_3
DICK *et al.* (1947)	α	4·46 MeV			1·42	1·20	(1·35)	1·31		1·40
BISTLINE (1948)	α	5·3 ,,	(1·00)							1·34
APPLEYARD (1949)	α	5·3 ,,					(1·35)		1·19	
HAEBERLI *et al.* (1953)	α	5·3 ,,	(1·00)		1·38	1·23		1·28		
VALENTINE and CURRAN (1952)	α	5·3 ,,	(1·00)	1·43	1·39	1·24	1·36			
SHARPE (1952)	α	5·16 ,,	(1·00)		1·38	1·25	1·35	1·30		
BORTNER and HURST (1953)	α	5·3 ,,	(1·00)	1·40	1·38	1·22	1·33	1·30		
JESSE and SADAUSKIS (1953)	α	5·3 ,,	(1·000)	1·375	1·386	1·231	1·345	1·307		1·37
,, ,, ,, ,,	α	~1·2 ,,	(1·000)		1·440		1·405	1·375		
Average	α	~5 ,,	(1·00)	1·40	1·39	1·23	1·35	1·30	1·19	1·37
BAKKER and SEGRÈ (1951)	p	340 ,,	(1·00)	1·38	1·31	1·23	1·30			
		Mean initial energy								
VALENTINE (1952)	e	2·8 keV	(1·00)	1·38	1·30					
,, ,,	e	5·7 ,,	(1·00)	1·41	1·33	1·19	1·30			
JESSE and SADAUSKIS (1955)	e	5·7 ,,	(1·00)	1·41	1·33	1·18	1·28	1·24		
HARDWICK (1954)	e	~ 4 ,,	(1·00)	1·37	1·32	1·17	1·29	1·24		
JESSE and SADAUSKIS (1955)	e	~ 17 ,,	(1·00)	1·38			1·30	1·25		
WEISS and BERNSTEIN (1955)	e	~200 ,,	0·97		1·33	1·18	(1·29)	1·25		
MUNSON (unpublished)	e	~300 ,,				1·19	(1·29)	1·25	1·08	
FAILLA and ROSSI (1954)	e				1·33	1·18	(1·29)	1·25		
Average	e		(1·00)	1·39	1·32	1·18	1·29	1·25	1·08	
W(gas)/W(argon)			(1·00)		1·333		1·285	1·240		
μ			(0·00)		0·15		0·21	0·18	0·33	

When values for argon were either not determined or were in doubt (see text), the mean values for air have been taken as the reference point (values in brackets).

On the whole the results of different observers are in good agreement. It will be seen that the average values of the ratio W(gas)/W(argon) for alpha particles are appreciably larger than those for electrons, except in the case of hydrogen. This suggests that in all the other gases W is dependent on the alpha particle energy, confirmation of this being provided by the observations of Jesse and Sadauskis (1953) (Table 18) with alpha particles of 1·2 MeV. When one fits equation (52) to their results for 1·2 and 5·3 MeV, the values of μ for nitrogen, carbon dioxide and air are found to be 0·15, 0·18 and 0·21 respectively, whilst the values of $W_\alpha(\infty)$ relative to W for argon are 1·333, 1·240, and 1·285. These are seen to differ by less than one per cent from the corresponding relative values of W_e. It will also be noted that there is good agreement between the relative values of W_e for hydrogen, nitrogen and air and those for 340 MeV protons. The initial speed of these protons was $95v_0$ and with $\mu = 0{\cdot}18$, $W(\infty)/W$ would be 0·996, so that a close agreement between the values of W for fast electrons and high energy protons is to be expected. For water vapour the value of μ given in Table 18 is derived from the measurements of Appleyard (1949) with alpha particles, and Munson (unpublished) with electrons on the assumption that $W_\alpha(\infty) = W_e$.

(v) *General Conclusions for Pure Gases*

After discussing their own recent results and those of other workers, Jesse and Sadauskis (1955) summarized their conclusions in the two following postulates.

(1) 'If in the relation $W_\alpha/W_e =$ constant for hydrogen and the noble gases, we assume this constant to be unity then W in these gases is the same both for beta and alpha particles throughout all ranges of energy for either so far measured by us' (i.e. Jesse and Sadauskis).

(2) 'In all other gases so far measured W_α/W_e is not found to be constant. The variation in the ratio seems to come from a variation of W_α with alpha particle energy. As the alpha particle energy increases this ratio approaches a constant value which again is probably unity.'

Jesse and Sadauskis were planning further experiments to prove or disprove these postulates, but in the meantime our examination of the data has persuaded us to accept them provisionally together with the following assumptions:

(3) In all gases other than the inert gases and hydrogen, the instantaneous value of the energy loss per ion pair $*W$ is dependent upon particle speed according to the relation

$$*W/W(\infty) = 1 + \mu\,(v_0/*v)$$

where μ is a dimensionless parameter, $v_0 \equiv e^2/\hbar$ and $*v$ is the particle velocity. μ increases very slowly with particle mass so that for ionizing particles whose masses lie between 1 and 19 (H = 1), one may assume that μ has the same value as for an alpha particle.

(4) The value of μ for all particles in argon even when containing small amounts of impurity is zero.

Although we consider that the values of W derived in this way are the best, alternative values based on the assumption that μ is really zero for all gases have also been used in our calculations (Tables 4 and 7). A comparison of these two values for W provides some indication of the uncertainty still attaching to this quantity.

(vi) *Ionization by Neutron Recoils*

If the elastic scattering of neutrons with atoms of type i is isotropic in centre of mass coordinates and the average energy loss per ion pair, W, is independent of the initial energy of the recoil particles ϵ_i, then from equations (1) and (2) the average number of ions produced by each recoil will be

$$\frac{\bar{\epsilon}_i}{W} = \frac{2A_i}{(1+A_i)^2} \cdot \frac{\epsilon}{W} \tag{53}$$

where $\bar{\epsilon}_i$ is the average energy of the recoils. On the other hand, if W is dependent upon the energy of the particle, it will change with the angle θ through which the neutron is scattered (centre of mass coordinates).

If $j(\theta)$ is the number of ions produced by a recoil ejected at the neutron scattering angle θ, the average ionization per recoil particle will be given by $\bar{j}$ where

$$\bar{j} = \tfrac{1}{2}\int_0^{\pi} j(\theta)\sin\theta\, d\theta. \tag{54}$$

Now

$$j(\theta) = \frac{2A_i\epsilon}{(1+A_i)^2} \cdot \frac{W(\infty)}{W} \cdot (1-\cos\theta) \tag{55}$$

where $W(\infty)/W$ is given by equation (52).

By integration of (55) with respect to θ, one finds the average ionization efficiency

$$\eta = 1 - \frac{4\sqrt{2}}{3}\left(\frac{\mu v_0}{v}\right) + 2\left(\frac{\mu v_0}{v}\right)^2 \times \left\{\left[1-\frac{1}{2}\left(\frac{\mu v_0}{v}\right)^2\right]\ln\left[1+\sqrt{2}\left(\frac{v}{\mu v_0}\right)\right] - \frac{1}{2} + \frac{1}{\sqrt{2}}\left(\frac{\mu v_0}{v}\right)\right\}. \tag{56}$$

The ionization efficiency given by this formula is slightly larger than that for a particle of initial energy ϵ_i and speed v found from equation (52) except at very low values of ϵ_i, but the difference does not exceed 0·03. The efficiencies given by (52) and (56) are plotted against $\mu v_0/v$ in Fig. 11.

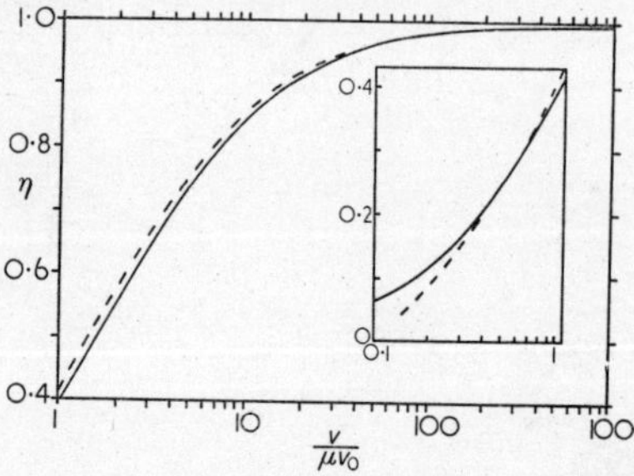

FIG. 11. Ionizing efficiency η as a function of $v/\mu v_0$. The full line applies to particles of initial speed v (equation 52), the broken line to neutron recoils of speed v corresponding to the average initial energy (equation 56).

When the neutron energy spectrum is continuous and there is a flux of $N(\epsilon)\,d\epsilon$ neutrons with energies between ϵ and $\epsilon+d\epsilon$, the number of ion pairs produced in the gas per sec per atom of type i is

$$\frac{2A_i}{(1+A_i)^2}\cdot\frac{1}{W(\infty)}\int_0^\infty \eta\epsilon\sigma_i(\epsilon)N(\epsilon)\,d\epsilon \tag{57}$$

where $\sigma_i(\epsilon)$ is the scattering cross section of atoms of type i for neutrons of energy ϵ and η is the ionization efficiency of the recoils given by equation (56). The average energy per ion pair can be found by dividing the R.H.S. of equation (14) by the expression (57).

(vii) *Energy per Ion Pair in Gas Mixtures*

The number of ions produced in a small mass of a gas exposed to ionizing particles is proportional to $P_i s_i/W_i$, where P_i is the gas pressure at a given fixed temperature, s_i is the molecular stopping power of the gas for the particles and W_i is the energy per ion pair. If other gases are added and no component in the resulting mixture interferes in any way with the ionization of the others, then the average energy per ion pair for the mixture, $\overline{W}$, will be given by

$$\frac{\Sigma P_i s_i}{\overline{W}} = \sum\left(\frac{P_i s_i}{W_i}\right). \tag{58}$$

The numbers of ions produced by alpha particles in binary mixtures of gases have been measured by Haeberli, Huber and Baldinger (1953), Valentine and Curran (1952) and Bortner and Hurst (1954), and deviations of a few per cent from the ionization calculated by equation (58) have been observed. Haeberli *et al.* interpreted such deviations as indicating that the energy per ion pair for delta rays is different from that for the primary alpha particles. Bortner and Hurst have pointed out that they could also be due to errors in the assumed values of stopping power.

When very small amounts of argon (0·13 per cent) were added to pure neon Jesse and Sadauskis (1952) found that W for alpha particles was almost as low as that for pure argon. This result was attributed to the ionization of argon atoms when in collision with neon atoms in excited metastable states, the ionization per collision having a high probability because the ionization potential of argon is very close to the energy of an excited neon atom. A similar effect was also found with pure helium to which a trace of neon had been added. Although these observations of Jesse and Sadauskis are of considerable intrinsic interest, they have no apparent bearing on the deviations from equation (58) which have been observed by others when the concentrations of the component gases were of the same order.

Valentine (1952) has measured the ionization produced by electrons from ^{37}A and ^{3}H in binary mixtures of argon with hydrogen and nitrogen and has found deviations of several per cent from the relation (58). The graphs of ionization current as a function of argon concentration using ^{37}A had somewhat different shapes from those obtained with electrons from ^{3}H, the differences in ionization current at a given argon concentration being nearly as large at some points as the deviation from the straight line given by (58). It is difficult to explain these findings in terms of the difference between the average energies of the electrons.

Munson (unpublished) has found that the ionization by secondary electrons from radium gamma rays in binary mixtures of the gases hydrogen, air, water vapour and carbon dioxide are in good agreement with those given by (58).

In view of the rather meagre and somewhat conflicting experimental evidence for mixtures of the gases used in the tissue chamber, the ionization due to neutron recoils and secondary electrons in this chamber has been calculated on the assumption that equation (58) is true. The results of these calculations appear in Tables 4 and 9.

17. SUMMARY

Tissue radiation doses in rads due to fast neutrons from uranium fission were estimated by measuring the ionization current in a homogeneous chamber filled with acetylene. The ionization due to slow neutrons and gamma radiation accompanying the fast neutrons was found by simultaneous measurements with two other chambers, one having copper electrodes and filled with boron trifluoride, the other with magnesium electrodes and filled with argon. Results obtained with the acetylene chamber were confirmed in some cases by observations with a homogeneous chamber having a composition nearly matching that of tissue.

The successful application of this method depended mainly upon three factors. Firstly, the energy absorption in tissue exposed to neutrons is approximately proportional to the ionization in the acetylene chamber at energies greater than 10^4 eV, whilst below 10 eV it is proportional to the ionization in the boron trifluoride chamber. Secondly, the relative ionizations in the three chambers due to gamma rays could be accurately calculated, since their energies (average 0·7 MeV) were in the range in which Compton scattering was the only important interaction process. Thirdly, the fluxes of slow neutrons were so small that the ionization currents generated by them in the acetylene and argon chambers were only of the order of one per cent of those due to fast neutrons and gamma rays.

It was shown that the ionization currents in the non-homogeneous chambers, when exposed to fast neutrons, would differ by less than one per cent from the currents in hypothetical homogeneous chambers filled with the same gases. Calculated corrections of a few per cent have been made to allow for attenuation of the radiations in the walls of the chambers.

Recent experimental evidence concerning the dependence upon speed of the ionizing efficiency of charged particles in gases has been reviewed. It was found that existing data for alpha particles can be adequately described in terms of an empirical relation with two adjustable parameters. This relation has been used to calculate the average energy per ion pair for neutron recoils in the ionization chambers. It appears that uncertainty in this quantity is probably the largest source of error ($\sim$ 10 per cent.) in the estimation of fast neutron dose for neutrons of energy below 1 MeV.

APPENDIX

Ionization Currents in Chambers Exposed to Slow Neutrons

The ionization current in a chamber irradiated by slow neutrons is caused by reactions such as (n, γ) and (n, α) with nuclei of the wall and gas, or by beta and gamma radiation from radioactive nuclei or by a combination of both.

The calculation of the ionization in the boron trifluoride chamber is particularly simple since the α particle and ^{7}Li recoil have ranges in the gas which are rather small compared with the chamber dimensions. From equations (8) and (12) the ionization rate in a very large chamber exposed to unit flux of slow neutrons would be

$$J = n_B \sigma_B \left(\frac{\epsilon_\alpha}{W_\alpha} + \frac{\epsilon_{Li}}{W_{Li}} \right) \tag{59}$$

where n_B is the number of boron atoms per gramme of gas ($= 8 \cdot 89 \, . \, 10^{21}$), σ_B is the reaction cross section ($= 854$ barns), ϵ_α ($= 1 \cdot 48$ MeV) and ϵ_{Li} ($= 0 \cdot 86$ MeV) are the initial kinetic energies of the α particle and ^{7}Li recoil, and W_α, W_{Li} are respectively the values of the energy dissipation per ion pair for these particles in boron trifluoride. The correction for the finite size of the chamber has been dealt with previously (Chap. II, §8 (i), p. 43), whilst the ionization contributions by gamma rays from ^{7}Li and from ^{66}Cu were found using the expressions given below. The available experimental data for the energy per ion pair in boron trifluoride are limited to alpha particles of about 5 MeV (Table 18) so that the value of W for ^{7}Li is unknown. The values of W have been calculated on the alternative assumptions:

(1) that $\mu = 0$ for both particles, and
(2) that $\mu = 0 \cdot 23$ for both particles

the latter being the average of the values for alpha particles in nitrogen, carbon dioxide, air and water (Table 18).

Beta and gamma radiation originating in the walls and gas fillings of the acetylene, magnesium-argon and tissue chambers under slow neutron irradiation lead to ionization within them. As each of these radiations may be produced in either the wall or gas, separate expressions are derived in the following sections to meet each case.

(1) *β Particles emitted from Chamber Wall*

Consider a chamber with a wall containing n_i nuclei g^{-1} of type i, each with a neutron activation cross section ${}_a\sigma_i$. The number of radioactive nuclei produced will be $n_i \, {}_a\sigma_i S$ g^{-1} sec^{-1} where S is the neutron flux. If the average energy of the β particles is $\bar{\epsilon}_\beta$, the rate of energy release in the wall at radioactive equilibrium is $n_i \, {}_a\sigma_i S \bar{\epsilon}_\beta$ MeV g^{-1} sec^{-1}. When the β particles lose only a small fraction of their energy in the gas and the thickness of the chamber wall exceeds the range of the fastest β particles, the ionization rate (ions g^{-1} sec^{-1}) in the gas is $n_i \, {}_a\sigma_i S \bar{\epsilon}_\beta \, 10^6 / W\rho$ where W is the average energy (eV) expended by the β particles in producing one pair of ions and ρ is the ratio of the mass stopping powers of the wall and gas.

(2) *β Particles emitted from Gas Atoms*

The number of ions formed by a single β particle emitted from a gas atom is equal to the product of the length of its track in the gas and the average specific ionization s along it. Since in general the points of origin of β particles will be uniformly distributed throughout the gas and the directions of emission will be random, the average track length l will be dependent upon the shape and size of the gas volume. In order to calculate the ionization rate, viz. $Sn_{i\ a}\sigma_i sl$ it is therefore necessary to find l for chambers of different shapes.

For a sphere, it can be readily shown that $l = 3a/4$ where a is the radius of the sphere. Those tracks which originate at the surface of the sphere have an average length of $a/2$ whilst those radiating from the centre have a length a. Thus the average track length for the whole sphere is the arithmetic mean of the values for the centre and the surface.

The only other figure for which similar calculations have been attempted is a cylinder of infinite length. The average lengths of tracks originating at the axis and at the surface are respectively $\pi a/2$ and a, where a is the radius. An exact value for the whole cylinder could not be found by simple integration and a solution by a more elaborate method did not appear worth while, but it is probable that it would be close to the arithmetic mean of $\pi a/2$ and a on the basis of the results for spheres. For cylinders of finite length with shapes similar to those of the ionization chambers used in this work, l is almost certainly within the limits $5a/4 \pm a/4$.

When a β particle emitted from a gas atom reaches the inner surface of the chamber wall, there is an appreciable probability that it will be scattered back into the gas, e.g. McInally and Neary (1953) found a 'reflection' coefficient of 0·27 for β particles from ^{32}P incident on a surface composed of light elements. The effective path length in the gas will therefore be increased by successive reflections, becoming for the sphere

$$\frac{3a}{4}+\frac{a}{2}(r+r^2+r^3\ldots) \quad \text{i.e.}\ \frac{a}{4}\cdot\frac{3-r}{1-r}$$

and for the cylinder

$$\frac{5a}{4}\pm\frac{a}{4}+a(r+r^2+r^3\ldots) \quad \text{i.e.}\ \frac{a}{4}\left(\frac{5-r}{1-r}\pm 1\right)$$

where the 'reflection' coefficient r is averaged over all angles of incidence and 'reflection'.

(3) Gamma Radiation from Chamber Wall

Gamma radiation from atoms of the chamber wall is partly absorbed in the wall giving rise to the emission of secondary electrons. If the average rate of energy absorption per unit volume of the wall over its inner surface is known, the ionization current can be found from Gray's relation (equation 12). In the case of a thick walled spherical chamber of internal radius a, external radius b and density Δ, the gamma ray energy flux G at the inner surface is given by

$$G = n_{i\,a}\sigma_i Sh\nu_i \Delta(b-a)\left(1+\frac{b+a}{2a}\ln\frac{b+a}{b-a}\right) \tag{60}$$

when one photon of energy $h\nu_i$ is emitted per neutron absorbed and gamma ray absorption in the wall is neglected. The ionization rate in the gas is then

$$J = GZ_g n_g s_g(\sigma_a+\tau)/_w W s_w. \tag{61}$$

When the chamber is in the form of a cylinder of internal and external radii a and b and is of infinite length, an exact expression for the ionization cannot be found. A numerical solution shows that when b/a has the values 1·01, 1·15, and 1·30, the ionization in an infinite cylinder exceeds that in a sphere of the same radius by the factors 1·50, 1·72 and 1·93 respectively. For cylindrical chambers of finite length these factors are somewhat smaller, e.g. for the magnesium and CH chambers of length $13a$, the corresponding factors are 1·47, 1·62, and 1·81 approximately. In practice, the presence of an axial electrode of length $2l$ and radius $b-a$, increases the ionization by 0·1 per cent, 4 per cent and 11 per cent when b/a has the values 1·01, 1·15 and 1·30 respectively.

(4) Gamma Radiation from Atoms of the Gas

It can be shown that the gamma ray energy flux at the surface of a sphere of gas activated by slow neutron irradiation is $\frac{1}{2}\delta San_{g\,a}\sigma_g h\nu_g$ where δ is the gas density, a is the radius, n_g the number of gas atoms per gramme, ${}_a\sigma_g$ is the reaction cross section of a gas atom and $h\nu_g$ the energy of the single photon which is assumed to result from the capture of one neutron. The ionization rate in the gas, by Gray's relation, is

$$\frac{\delta}{2}San_g^{2}\,{}_a\sigma_g h\nu_g(\sigma_a+\tau)_w Z_g s_g/Ws_w \tag{62}$$

With a homogeneous chamber the ratio of the ionization due to gamma radiation from the gas to that due to radiation from the wall is approximately

$$\frac{1}{2}\frac{\delta}{\Delta}\cdot\frac{n_g}{n_i}\cdot\frac{{}_a\sigma_g}{{}_a\sigma_i}\cdot\frac{a}{(b-a)}\cdot\frac{1}{\left(1+\frac{b+a}{2a}\ln\frac{b+a}{b-a}\right)} \tag{63}$$

and in practice is usually so small that it may be neglected.

(5) *Gamma Radiation from Brass Clamping Rings*

Brass clamping rings (Fig. 7) were fitted to four of the chambers and these emitted gamma radiation which arose partly from neutron capture and partly from the radioactive products such as ^{66}Cu. Since the cross sections of some of the stable isotopes of Zn and Cu are not known, it is not possible to calculate the gamma ray emission from brass with any precision. The ionization in the chamber was estimated by making the simplifying assumptions that the metal of the ring was concentrated into an infinitely thin ring and that the gas of the chamber was compressed along the axis of this ring.

REFERENCES

ADAIR, R. K., *Rev. Mod. Phys.*, 1950, **22**, 249.
APPLEYARD, R. K., *Nature* (*London*), 1949, **164**, 838.
ARON, W. A., HOFFMAN, B. G., and WILLIAMS, F. C., U.S. Atomic Energy Commission Report AECU–663, 1949.
BAKKER, C. J., and SEGRÈ, E., *Phys. Rev.*, 1950, **77**, 782.
BARSCHALL, H. H., *Rev. Mod. Phys.*, 1952, **24**, 120.
BEHRENS, D. J., A.E.R.E. Harwell Memorandum AERE/TM6, 1948.
BISTLINE, J. A., *Rev. Sci. Instr.*, 1948, **19**, 482.
BORTNER, T. E., and HURST, G. S., *Phys. Rev.*, 1953, **90**, 160.
BRETSCHER, E., and FRENCH, A. P., Report BR517, 1944.
BREUNIG, E., *Ann. Phys. Lpz.*, 1936, **25**, 467.
BNL–325, Brookhaven National Laboratory publication "Neutron Cross Sections", 1955 (ed. D. J. HUGHES and J. A. HARVEY).
CAPLEHORN, W. F., and RUNDLE, G. P., *Proc. Phys. Soc.* A, 1951, **64**, 546.
CORMACK, D. V., and JOHNS, H. E., *Brit. J. Radiol.*, 1952, **25**, 369.
CRANSHAW, T. E., and HARVEY, J. A., *Canad. J. Res.* A, 1948, **26**, 243.
DAINTY, J., Chalk River Report CRM–482, 1950.
DAVISSON, C. M., and EVANS, R. D., *Rev. Mod. Phys.*, 1952, **24**, 79.
DE JUREN, L. A., and ROSENWASSER, H., *Phys. Rev.*, 1954, **93**, 831.
DICK, L., FALK-VAIRANT, P., and ROSSEL, J., *Helv. Phys. Acta*, 1947, **20**, 357.
ELLIS, C. D., and ASTON, G. H., *Proc. Roy. Soc.* A, 1930, **129**, 180.
ERSKINE, G. A., *Proc. Roy. Soc.* A, 1954, **224**, 362.
FAILLA, G., and ROSSI, H. H., U.S. Atomic Energy Commission Report, NYO 4582, 1954.
FANO, U., *Phys. Rev.*, 1946, **70**, 44.

FREUND, L., *Ann. Phys. Lpz.*, 1935, **22**, 748.
GERBES, W., *Ann. Phys. Lpz.*, 1935, **23**, 648.
GERBES, W., *Ann. Phys. Lpz.*, 1937, **30**, 169.
GRAY, L. H., *Proc. Roy. Soc.* A, 1929, **122**, 648.
GRAY, L. H., *Proc. Roy. Soc.* A, 1936, **156**, 578.
GRAY, L. H., *Proc. Camb. Phil. Soc.*, 1944, **40**, 72.
HAEBERLI, W., HUBER, P., and BALDINGER, E., *Helv. Phys. Acta*, 1953, **26**, 145.
HAMOUDA, I., and MONTMOLLIN, G. DE, *Helv. Phys. Acta*, 1952, **25**, 107.
HANNA, G. C., *Phys. Rev.*, 1950, **80**, 530.
HATFIELD, T. N., LOCKENITZ, A. E., and COLBY, M. Y., *J. Franklin Inst.*, 1949, **247**, 133.
HARDWICK, T. J. (quoted by Erskine, G. A., *Proc. Roy. Soc.* A, 1954, **224**, 363).
HOLLANDER, J. M., PERLMAN, I., and SEABORG, G. T., *Rev. Mod. Phys.*, 1953, **25**, 469.
HORNYAK, W. F., LAURITSEN, T., MORRISON, P., and FOWLER, W. A., *Rev. Mod. Phys.*, 1950, **22**, 291.
HURST, G. S., *Brit. J. Radiol.*, 1954, **27**, 353.
JAHNKE, E., and EMDE, F., *Tables of Functions with Formulae and Curves*, 1945, Dover Publications, New York.
JESSE, W. P., FORSTAT, H., and SADAUSKIS, J., *Phys. Rev.*, 1950, **77**, 782.
JESSE, W. P., and SADAUSKIS, J., *Phys. Rev.*, 1950, **78**, 1.
JESSE, W. P., and SADAUSKIS, J., *Phys. Rev.*, 1952, **88**, 417.
JESSE, W. P., and SADAUSKIS, J., *Phys. Rev.*, 1953, **90**, 1120.
JESSE, W. P., and SADAUSKIS, J., *Phys. Rev.*, 1955, **97**, 1668.
LIVINGSTON, M. S., and BETHE, H. A., *Rev. Mod. Phys.*, 1937, **9**, 261.
MCINALLY, M., and NEARY, G. J., *Brit. J. Radiol.*, 1953, **26**, 539.
MILLS, R. G., UCRL Report Number 1815, 1952.
NEARY, G. J., MUNSON, R. J., and MOLE, R. H., *Nature* (*London*), 1953, **171**, 256.
NICODEMUS, D. B., Thesis, Stanford University, 1946.
PIGGE, H., *Ann. Phys. Lpz.*, 1934, **20**, 233.
Recommendations of the International Commission on Radiological Units, Copenhagen, 1953.
Recommendations of the International Commission on Radiological Protection, *Brit. J. Radiol. Suppl.* No. 6, 1955.
RHODES, J., FRANZEN, W., and STEPHENS, W. E., *Phys. Rev.*, 1952, **87**, 141.
ROSSI, H. H., and FAILLA, G., *Nucleonics*, 1956, **14**, No. 2, 32.
Science and Engineering of Nuclear Power, Vol. I, 1947 (ed. CLARK GOODMAN), Addison-Wesley Press Inc., Cambridge, Mass.
SHARPE, J., *Proc. Phys. Soc.*, A, 1952, **65**, 859.
STONE, W. G., and COCHRAN, L. W., *Phys. Rev.*, 1954, **95**, 304.
TUNNICLIFFE, P. R., and WARD, A. G., *Proc. Phys. Soc.* A, 1952, **65**, 233.
VALENTINE, J. M., *Proc. Roy. Soc.* A, 1952, **211**, 75.
VALENTINE, J. M., and CURRAN, S. C., *Phil. Mag.*, 1952, **42**, 964.
WARSHAW, S. D., *Phys. Rev.*, 1949, **76**, 1759.
WATT, B. E., *Phys. Rev.*, 1952, **87**, 1037.
WEISS, J., and BERNSTEIN, W., *Phys. Rev.*, 1955, **98**, 1828.

CHAPTER III

RESULTS OF FAST NEUTRON IRRADIATION

1. RECORDS OF DOSAGE AND ENVIRONMENT

(i) *Dosage*

THE dose per week could not be maintained exactly constant because of unavoidable variations in the pile operating programme. Any excess or deficiency in a given week was normally corrected in the following week by varying the time during which the shutters were

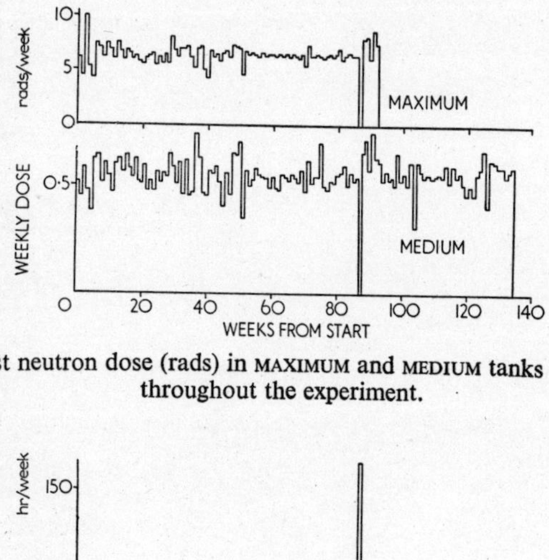

FIG. 12. Fast neutron dose (rads) in MAXIMUM and MEDIUM tanks week by week throughout the experiment.

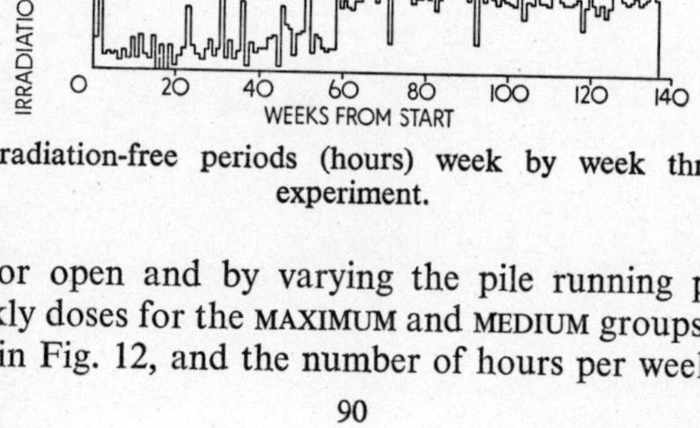

FIG. 13. Irradiation-free periods (hours) week by week throughout the experiment.

kept shut or open and by varying the pile running power. The actual weekly doses for the MAXIMUM and MEDIUM groups of animals are shown in Fig. 12, and the number of hours per week free from irradiation in Fig. 13. The mean weekly doses and irradiation free period for all tanks are given in Table 19.

Besides the random errors of measurement shown in Table 19 there were also systematic errors affecting all groups which are estimated at about 13 per cent (Chap. II, §12 (i), p. 55). There was also a variation of dose rate over the area of each tank, amounting to about ±10 per cent of the mean (Chap. I, §9, p. 12). The animals in a given tank were not systematically shuffled around, but no correlation of radiation effects with position originally occupied in the tank was discovered.

TABLE 19

Mean weekly dose rates and irradiation-free time

Group	MAXIMUM	MEDIUM	MINIMUM	GAMMA
Mean neutron dose rate rads/wk.	6·41±0·13	0·540±0·032	0·191±0·030	0·084±0·028
Highest weekly dose	9·95	0·737	0·282	0·140
Lowest weekly dose†	4·10	0·314	0·092	0·051
Standard deviation of weekly neutron doses	1·07	0·086	0·033	0·019
Mean gamma dose rate r/wk.	1·64±0·12	0·843±0·017	0·980±0·014	0·668±0·013
Mean weekly radiation-free hours	24·1	26·8	27·1	27·2

† Except for one week when the pile was shut down completely (Figs. 12 and 13).

The mean doses are given to three figures although the third figure is not reliable. The errors shown are the random errors of measurement (Table 1). The systematic errors are considered in Chap. II, § 12, p. 52. The doses quoted in a previous publication (Neary, Munson and Mole, 1953) have since been revised (Chap. II, § 7 (i), p. 41).

(ii) *Environmental Temperature*

The natural temperature level in the experimental tanks was very stable around 70°F because these tanks were sunk into the large concrete shield of the pile. The CONTROL tank, however, was more exposed, and its temperature would have fluctuated appreciably. This tank was therefore surrounded by a jacket through which air was circulated from an air-conditioning plant and the temperature was thermostatically maintained at 70°F. Alarm circuits were provided so that if any fault should occur in the air-conditioning plant, warning bells and lights would operate when the temperature in the tank deviated up or down by more than 5 degrees F.

Maximum and minimum thermometers were read daily in the CONTROL tank and in the GAMMA tank but these were replaced after about six months by continuously recording thermographs. The temperature in the GAMMA tank was always very close to the temperatures in the three other experimental tanks. The variation during any single 24-hour period was very small and the weekly maximum and minimum temperatures in the GAMMA and CONTROL tanks have been analysed; some relevant data are summarized in Table 20.

After the first year and a half (Table 20, First Period) there was an increase of approximately 2 degrees F in the mean temperature of the experimental tanks (Table 20, Second Period). The overall mean temperature for the whole experiment was 70·7°F, the same as that of the CONTROL tank. The mean temperature of the temperature-controlled box used in the second period for one day per week to house the animals from the experimental tanks was 71·0°F, with a standard deviation 1·3 degrees, and was thus within half a degree of the mean temperature in the CONTROL tank.

TABLE 20

Environmental temperatures (degrees F)

	GAMMA tank			CONTROL tank
	First period (first 18 months)	Second period (last 14 months)	Mean of 1 and 2	
Mean weekly maximum temperature	71·0	72·9	71·9	72·2
Standard deviation	2·2	2·5	3·6	2·7
Mean weekly minimum temperature	68·5	70·4	69·5	69·2
Standard deviation	2·6	2·1	3·5	2·1

2. EFFECTS OF CONTINUED EXPOSURE TO DEATH

(i) *Survival Times*

The day of death of each animal is recorded in Tables 21 and 22. The survival time was measured from the beginning of the experiment on 1st January 1951 when the mean age was 13 weeks, and was rarely in error by more than one day.

Before undertaking an analysis of these survival times it was necessary to exclude fourteen animals which escaped or were accidentally killed. They are specially indicated in Tables 21 and 22, and there can be no doubt of the validity of their exclusion. In addition eleven other mice have been excluded which died during the first 12½ months. They came from three cages (one MEDIUM male, two CONTROL female) where from three to four mice died

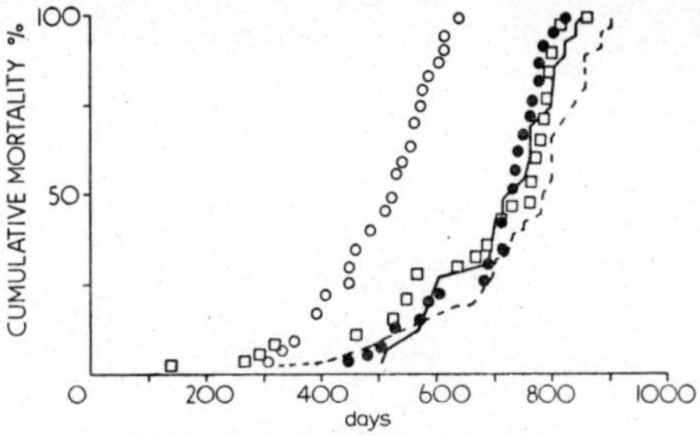

FIG. 14. Cumulative mortality (per cent) for male CBA mice and duration of irradiation by fast neutrons (days).

○ MAXIMUM tank, fast neutrons 6·4 rads weekly
● MEDIUM tank, fast neutrons 0·54 rads weekly
□ MINIMUM tank, fast neutrons 0·19 rads weekly

The cumulative mortality in the GAMMA tank is shown by a continuous line, in the CONTROL tank by the broken line. Approximately every other death has been plotted in order not to show too many points and thus obscure comparisons where the different exposure groups almost overlap. A few animals have been omitted from the MEDIUM tank curve (see text).

within 48 hours of each other for no apparent reason. Their exclusion is not arbitrary since the distribution of deaths within all other cages was random. These mice are also specially indicated in Tables 21 and 22 so that, if desired, they may be included in any analysis of our data by others.

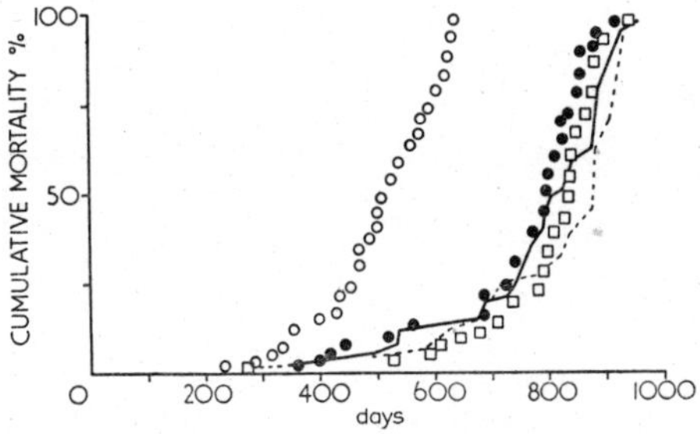

FIG. 15. Cumulative mortality (per cent) for female CBA mice and duration of irradiation by fast neutrons (days)

Symbols and plotting as in Fig. 14. A few animals have been omitted from the CONTROL tank curve (see text).

The cumulative mortality data are shown in Figs. 14 and 15, and the mean survival times for each irradiation group and sex in Table 23.

Gross effects were seen in the MAXIMUM tank where the mean survival time was shortened by a third. In the MEDIUM tank the mean survival time was shortened by less than ten per cent, the exact figure depending on what baseline is used for the comparison (see subsequent discussion).

TABLE 23

Mean survival times

Group	Sex	Number of animals		Mean survival time (days)	Standard deviation	Standard error of mean
		Initial	Analysed			
MAXIMUM	Male	50	50	499·6	89·8	12·7
	Female	50	50	510·8	100·9	14·3
MEDIUM	Male	49	40	703·7	98·8	15·6
	Female	50	49	758·1	134·7	19·2
MINIMUM	Male	50	49	676·2	165·5	23·6
	Female	50	49	802·9	115·6	16·5
GAMMA	Male	49	47	714·0	102·4	14·9
	Female	50	50	786·3	140·9	19·9
CONTROL	Male	49	47	742·9	137·2	20·0
	Female	50	41	818·1	139·7	21·8

In each group except the MAXIMUM, the mean survival time of the female animals was significantly greater (at the 5 per cent level) than those of the males. There was a general trend towards shorter mean survival times with increasing dose levels. There were significant differences between the MAXIMUM and all other groups for both males and females; and between the MINIMUM and CONTROL male groups, and MEDIUM and CONTROL female groups. The combined significance for males and females was calculated and differences significant at the 5 per cent level were found only between the MAXIMUM and all other groups; and between the MEDIUM and CONTROL groups.

The mortality curves get steeper the greater the age (Figs. 14 and 15), as is found also in standard life tables for human populations; their shape did not correspond to a normal distribution. The shapes of all the curves were similar, but from a general inspection there appeared to be more early deaths (i.e. early relative to mean survival time) in the lower dose groups, a point which is examined further below. In order to exclude these early deaths, the data for animals between the 30 per cent and 100 per cent mortality levels were also analysed (Table 24).

TABLE 24

Mean survival times, 30 to 100 per cent mortality

Group	Sex	Number of animals	Mean survival time (days)	Standard deviation	Standard error of mean
MAXIMUM	Male	35	549·6	49·6	8·4
	Female	35	565·0	54·0	9·1
MEDIUM	Male	27	758·5	32·6	6·2
	Female	34	829·4	41·5	7·1
MINIMUM	Male	34	770·2	45·4	7·8
	Female	34	859·2	34·0	5·8
GAMMA	Male	34	770·1	51·5	8·8
	Female	35	859·1	58·0	10·1
CONTROL	Male	33	817·3	55·0	9·6
	Female	29	891·9	38·2	7·1

The sex difference in survival, noted above, was also shown in these data, and was significant at the 5 per cent level in all groups except the MAXIMUM. The change in mean survival time with increasing dose was more regular and there were significant differences between more of the dose levels than for the complete data. Thus for males, there were significant differences not only between the MAXIMUM and all other groups, but also between the CONTROL and all other groups; for females, not only between the MAXIMUM and all other groups, but also between the MEDIUM and all other groups, and the CONTROL and all other groups. The combined data for males and females showed differences significant at the 5 per cent level between the MAXIMUM and all other groups, the MEDIUM and all other groups, the CONTROL and all other groups.

Although not all the differences in mean survival time (M.S.T.) between the groups were statistically significant (at the 5 per cent level), it is of interest to examine the shortening of M.S.T. in relation to (a) dose rate (b) mean accumulated dose. For this purpose the complete data (0–100 per cent mortality) for the males and females have been averaged (Table 25).

TABLE 25

Shortening of mean survival time relative to CONTROL *group (sexes averaged) complete data*

Group	Dose per week		M.S.T.	Shortening	
	Neutron	Gamma	(days)	(days)	(per cent)
MAXIMUM	6·41 rads	1·64 r	505·5	275·0	35
MEDIUM	0·54 rads	0·84 r	730·9	49·6	6
MINIMUM	0·19 rads	0·98 r	739·6	40·9	5
GAMMA	0·084 rads	0·67 r	750·2	30·3	4
CONTROL	0	0	780·5	—	

Allowance must be made for the dose due to gamma radiation, and this has been done by assuming alternative possible values of the relative biological efficiency (r.b.e.) for neutrons, namely 5 and ∞. Effective neutron dose rates were thus calculated, from which effective neutron doses accumulated in the mean survival times were obtained. The observed shortening of M.S.T. is plotted against dose rate and against dose in Fig. 16 (a) and (b), for r.b.e. = 5 and

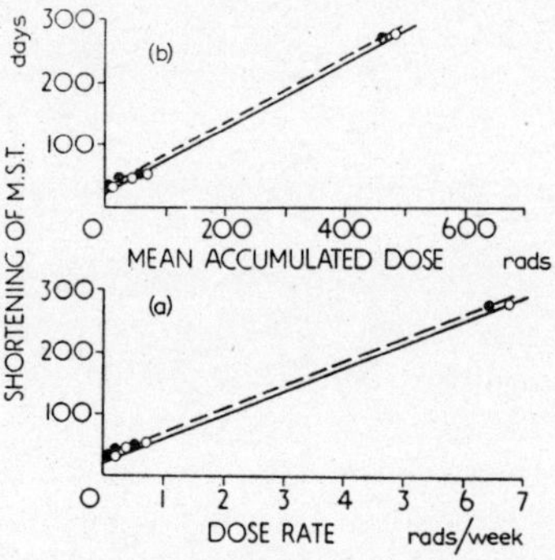

FIG. 16. Shortening of mean survival time (sexes averaged) as a function of (a) dose rate (b) mean accumulated dose.

—o——o— assuming r.b.e. is 5

-●--● - assuming r.b.e. is infinitely large

for r.b.e. = ∞. In each case a straight line may be drawn through the points. When extrapolated to zero dose rate or dose, the line indicates a positive shortening, implying that the environmental conditions *per se* in the experimental tanks were slightly less favourable than in the CONTROL tank; the magnitude of this effect is about 25 days. The parameters of the lines are given in Table 26; the slope depends only slightly on the figure assumed for the r.b.e. in evaluating the neutron equivalent of the gamma radiation because the gamma contribution is approximately the same in the different groups, except in the MAXIMUM where it is small relative to the neutron level.

TABLE 26

Regression line parameters for shortening of mean survival time, complete data

	Dose-rate		Dose	
R.B.E.	5	∞	5	∞
Slope	37 days/rad/wk	38 days/rad/wk	0·53 days/rad	0·54 days/rad
Intercept (days)	24	30	17	25

The shortening of 38 days for a dose rate of 1 rad/week may be compared with the figure 49 days* obtained for CF_1 mice by Henshaw *et al.* (1946), and 31 days for Swiss mice by Evans (1948). The data of Lorenz *et al.* (1954) for LAF_1 mice indicated 4 days' shortening for a gamma dose rate of 1 r/week. In terms of accumulated dose our figure of 0·54 days per rad may be compared with that of Lorenz *et al.* (1954) of 0·046 days per roentgen.

The data for animals between 30 and 100 per cent mortality may be treated similarly, and the resulting parameters are given in Table 27; they are not essentially different from those derived from the complete data.

TABLE 27

Regression line parameters for shortening of mean survival time, 30—100 *per cent mortality*

	Dose-rate		Dose	
R.B.E.	5	∞	5	∞
Slope	39 days/rad/wk	40 days/rad/wk	0·52 days/rad	0·52 days/rad
Intercept (days)	30	40	23	30

Analysis of Mortality

The relationship between the mortality curves is next examined in more detail. Two hypotheses will be considered, the first that

* Initial slope

radiation acts independently of the various other causes of death and thus superimposes an excess mortality upon that observed for unirradiated animals. The second is suggested by the fact that on casual inspection the curves are of the same shape; the effect of radiation may be merely to displace a mortality curve backwards along the time axis, making the deaths of all animals of a given irradiation level earlier by a certain amount.

Hypothesis of Excess Mortality

The hypothetical percentage mortality due to radiation alone is obtained by Abbott's formula and is equal to the difference between the observed mortalities in the experimental and control groups expressed as a percentage of the surviving fraction in the control group at that time. These excess mortalities expressed as probits were plotted against time. The male and female MAXIMUM groups each gave moderately straight lines, corresponding to approximately normal distributions. The probit plots for the MEDIUM and MINIMUM groups for both sexes approximated only roughly to straight lines after an initial 10 or 15 per cent mortality. Deaths before this point were straggled out very irregularly. This analysis thus suggests that there were two different modes of radiation death. The later straight parts of the probit plots were not all of the same slope, being steeper the lower the dose rate. The hypothesis of excess mortality does not seem to reveal any obvious regularities underlying the data. The probit plots of the two GAMMA groups were even less regular than those of the MEDIUM and MINIMUM, and it is scarcely justifiable to regard any portion of them as a straight line.

There are general grounds for preferring a comparison between an irradiated group and a GAMMA group rather than a CONTROL group, because of the closer correspondence between their environmental factors, e.g. small temperature variations, and the transfer from the normal experimental tanks to an irradiation-free temperature-controlled box for one day per week after the first year of the experiment. According to the analysis above, environmental differences between the CONTROL and the experimental tanks were responsible for a 20 to 30 day difference in life expectation. When the comparison was made with the GAMMA group, the probit plots for the MAXIMUM groups were scarcely changed, and those for the MEDIUM groups were not improved; those for the MINIMUM groups were very irregular.

Hypothesis of Premature Ageing

The underlying idea in this hypothesis is that radiation in some way causes the natural processes leading to death to come into play earlier, but that these processes once initiated are not thereafter accelerated. The reason for adopting this viewpoint was that the terminal portions of the mortality curves were not steeper for the high than for the low dose groups (see below), and so the whole time scale was not just contracted. The curves in fact seemed to be merely displaced along the time axis to the left, as would be expected if the early part of the time scale where mortality is very small were contracted, but not that part where deaths are occurring.

A corollary of this hypothesis is that the relative frequency of the various causes of death should be about the same in irradiated as in unirradiated animals; and further, that the effect of the radiation after mortality has become appreciable should be comparatively slight. The pathological findings (Chap. III, §2 (iii), p. 107) are roughly consistent with the first of these conclusions, so far as the broad classification for the various causes of death goes, but in the detailed classification, and in the timing of deaths, differences between the various groups were observed. The second of the two deductions agrees with the data presented later (Chap. III, §3 (iv), p. 140) on the shortening of life by limited periods of chronic irradiation, and with other data of Mole (1955) showing that the later part of a period of chronic irradiation may be largely wasted as far as its effect on shortening of life is concerned.

There is no unique method of testing the proposition that the rising parts of the mortality curves are all essentially of the same shape within the limits of statistical variation. First, it will be demonstrated that the curves for the MAXIMUM groups do not rise as steeply as would be expected if they were derived from the unirradiated groups by an overall contraction of the time scale. A convenient measure of the slope is afforded by the reciprocal of the standard deviation of survival time for the 30–100 per cent data. The comparison is made between the MAXIMUM group and the average of the MINIMUM, GAMMA and CONTROL groups for each sex separately. In order to superimpose the mean survival times of the average of the low dose curve and the MAXIMUM curve, the time scale for the former would have to be contracted in the ratio 0·70 for males and 0·64 for females. If the MAXIMUM curves were a simple contraction of the low dose curves the slopes of the former should therefore be $1/0{\cdot}70 = 1{\cdot}43$ and $1/0{\cdot}64 = 1{\cdot}56$ times as great as the slopes of the latter for males and females respectively. The observed slopes, however, were in the ratio 1·02 and 0·81, so that the MAXIMUM curves were certainly no steeper than the low dose curves.

As a next step, the curves for the five groups of male animals were plotted together, each about its own mean survival time as origin; the same was done for the female groups. It was then clear that in each case, the five different groups were fairly closely superimposed. A mean mortality curve for each sex was then derived by taking the mean of times for successive percentage mortalities in each group in steps of 2 per cent (since there were approximately 50 animals in each group). The deviations of the actual times of death of animals in a given group were read from the mean curve, and the root mean square value was calculated. It is clear that this standard deviation must be at least of the order of the standard error in the group's mean survival time (for this latter determines the overall position of the whole curve) and in fact should be about $\sqrt{(4/5)}$ of the latter. Thus a value of the observed standard deviation less than about twice $\sqrt{(4/5)}$ the standard error of mean survival times would imply that the shape of the curve for the particular group did not differ significantly from the mean curve. The figures for this comparison are given in Tables 28 and 29.

TABLE 28

Comparison with mean mortality curve, males

Group	MAXIMUM	MEDIUM	MINIMUM	GAMMA	CONTROL
Standard deviation from mean curve (days)	33·2	24·7	53·2	26·8	25·1
Limit of expected deviation (days)	22·2	27·3	41·3	26·0	35·0

TABLE 29

Comparison with mean mortality curve, females

Group	MAXIMUM	MEDIUM	MINIMUM	GAMMA	CONTROL
Standard deviation from mean curve (days)	35·4	21·5	27·4	21·0	27·5
Limit of expected deviation (days)	25·0	33·6	28·9	36·8	38·2

The statistical significance of the deviations larger than expected in the male MAXIMUM and MINIMUM and the female MAXIMUM groups is not obvious. From an inspection of the curves, it seemed that the early deaths were the main cause of difference between the groups. The shape of a limited portion of the mortality curves was therefore compared, choosing arbitrarily the portion from 30 per cent mortality onwards. It is implied in such a treatment of the data that there were comparable numbers of 'early' deaths in all groups, and that only their timing differed, that is timing relative to the groups mean survival time; in other words, deaths occurring by some particular mechanism at the same age equally in all groups, would in terms of the present analysis be 'earlier' in the longer lived groups. For the limited mortality data (30 to 100 per cent) the curves were superimposed as above, taking the mean survival time for each one as origin, and the mean curve was derived. The standard deviations and expected limits are given in Tables 30 and 31.

TABLE 30

Comparison with mean curve, males, 30–100 *per cent mortality*

Group	MAXIMUM	MEDIUM	MINIMUM	GAMMA	CONTROL
Standard deviation from mean curve (days)	6·1	16·4	11·5	8·6	10·2
Limit of expected deviation (days)	14·7	10·9	13·6	15·4	16·8

TABLE 31

Comparison with mean curve, females, 30–100 *per cent mortality*

Group	MAXIMUM	MEDIUM	MINIMUM	GAMMA	CONTROL
Standard deviation from mean curve (days)	11·7	6·7	12·7	15·3	10·5
Limit of expected deviation (days)	15·9	12·8	10·2	17·7	12·4

There is now only one group, the male MEDIUM, which falls appreciably outside the expected limit. It is concluded that there is no real difference in the shape of the later portions of the mortality curves, and, by implication, that the modes of death are the same over this range for the different groups.

The similarity of shape of the mortality curves may also be examined by a comparison of their standard deviations. The latter may be compared by means of the variance ratio test, though a precise test of significance is not possible because the samples are not normally distributed. It may first be noted that the sex difference in the MAXIMUM, MEDIUM, and CONTROL groups is not significant (at the 5 per cent level). For the male animals there is no significant difference between the standard deviations of the MAXIMUM, MEDIUM and GAMMA groups or between the MINIMUM and CONTROL groups. For the females, the same is true of the MAXIMUM and MINIMUM groups, and of the MEDIUM, MINIMUM, GAMMA and CONTROL groups.

For large samples of nearly equal numbers, the statistic z is distributed approximately normally about a mean of zero with a standard deviation $\sqrt{(1/n)}$, where $(n+1)$ is the number in the sample. n for these groups is about 46 and there is thus a 5 per cent chance that z should lie outside the range $\pm 0{\cdot}289$, i.e. that the ratio of standard deviations should exceed 1.335 either way. Now the average of the standard deviations of all groups for both sexes is 122·5 days and so any value within the limit 92 and 164 would not differ significantly from a value around 122·5. On this criterion, only the MAXIMUM male group (Table 23) falls outside the expected limits, and then only by a small margin.

If the 30–100 per cent mortality data only are considered, a z test shows that there is no significant difference between the male MAXIMUM, MINIMUM, GAMMA and CONTROL groups. For females, there is no significant difference between the MAXIMUM, MEDIUM, and GAMMA groups, or between the MEDIUM, MINIMUM and CONTROL groups. The average value of the standard deviation for all groups is 46·0 days, and by similar reasoning to that above, actual values between 33 and 64 days may be expected; these limits include all the groups (Table 24).

Another approximate argument is that the standard deviation of a large sample n is distributed nearly normally, with a standard deviation $\sigma/\sqrt{(2n)}$. For the complete mortality data, the estimate of σ is, as above, 122·5 days, and therefore values within the limits 98 to 147 may be expected with a 95 per cent probability; only the male MAXIMUM and MINIMUM groups (Table 23) fall outside these limits. For the 30–100 per cent data, the corresponding limits are 35 to 57; only the male MEDIUM and female GAMMA groups (Table 24) fall just outside.

Thus by the approximate application of a variety of statistical tests it has been shown that the mortality data are compatible with the hypothesis of premature ageing stated above. The effect of chronic whole body irradiation is to shorten the time during which ultimately lethal processes are initiated without altering the rate of dying when once deaths begin to occur.

The data of Lorenz *et al.* (1954) on survival of mice under irradiation by gamma rays (Table 32) showed a much more systematic trend towards smaller standard deviations of M.S.T. for higher dose levels than was observed in our neutron-irradiated mice over a biologically comparable range of dose levels.

The expected standard deviation of the standard deviation of survival time is about 13·8 days so that values within the range 107 to 163 could be expected. The 0,0·11 and 8·8 r/day groups fall outside these limits, the latter by a considerable margin. It would

TABLE 32

Standard deviation of mean survival time, data of Lorenz et al. (1954), *for gamma irradiation*

Daily dose (r/day)	Number of animals	Standard deviation (days)
0	59	176·5
0·11	45	174·1
1·1	48	138·4
2·2	47	137·0
4·4	48	110·8
8·8	45	73·8
Mean	48·7	135·1

be expected that above a certain dose rate, the standard deviation of survival time must decrease as the dose rate increases. Within the range of our experiment however, the simple hypothesis of premature ageing represents our data reasonably well, particularly if early deaths are excluded.

(ii) *Body Weight*

Each mouse was weighed ten days before the start of the experiment and at weekly intervals thereafter. The initial distribution of weights is shown in Fig. 17, and is normal except for 2 per cent of animals which were underweight (less than the Mean $-3\times$SD).

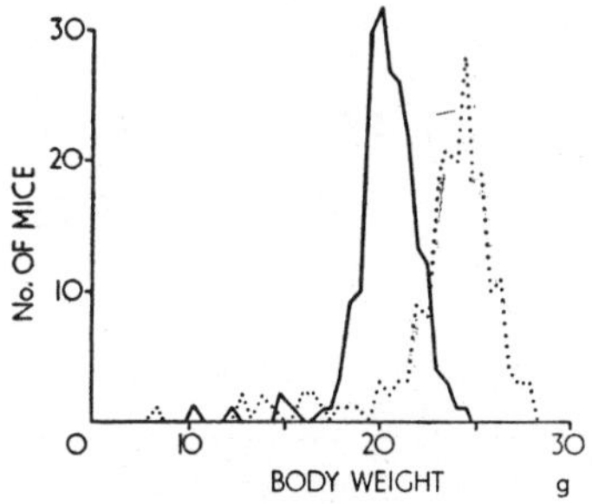

FIG. 17. Distribution of body weight (g) before the start of irradiation.
Males, dotted line
Females, continuous line

The mean monthly weights of males and females are shown separately in Figs. 18 and 19. There was a clear sex difference in growth rate but no effect of radiation except possibly for the female MAXIMUM group. The maximum weight was slightly less in the animals in the MAXIMUM tank, than in the other groups, 5 per cent less in males and 8 per cent less in females. The small differences in maximum weight between the other groups were due almost entirely to the few underweight mice.

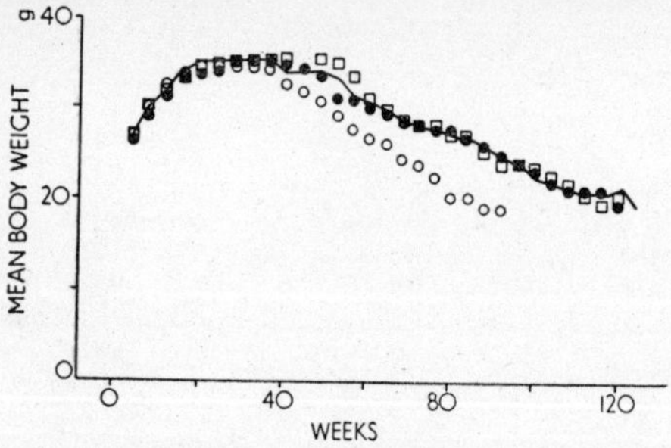

FIG. 18. Mean body weight (g) of male CBA mice during chronic irradiation by fast neutrons

Each point is a four-week average

○ MAXIMUM tank, fast neutrons 6·4 rads weekly
● MEDIUM tank, fast neutrons 0·57 rads weekly
□ MINIMUM tank, fast neutrons 0·19 rads weekly
— GAMMA tank

After 36 weeks the weight of both males and females in the MAXIMUM tank began suddenly to fall. This was not due to a fall in weight of a few individuals but a to general decrease in all the mice.

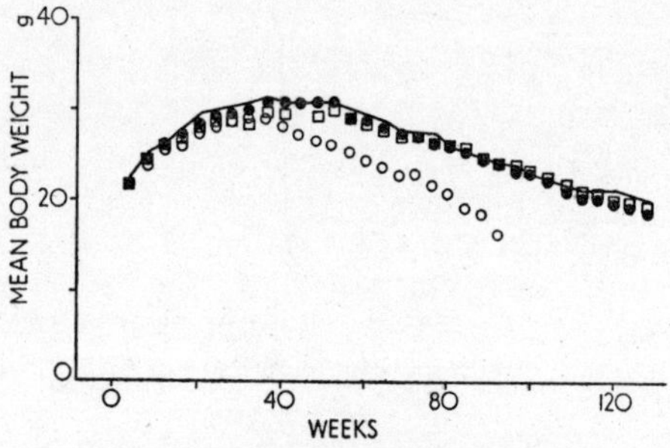

FIG. 19. Mean body weight (g) of female CBA mice during chronic irradiation by fast neutrons

Each point is a four-week average

Symbols as in Fig. 18

A similar but initially more gradual loss in weight occurred later and simultaneously in the other tanks; there was no real difference at any time between the MEDIUM tank and the MINIMUM and GAMMA tanks. In all tanks the loss in weight preceded the onset of an increased death rate.

As already mentioned (Chap. I, §7, p. 9), additional mice were placed in the irradiation tanks in cages half the standard size. These mice were also weighed weekly and their growth rate is shown in Fig. 20 compared with mice in standard cages. Although the cubic capacity of cage and floor area per mouse was the same in each type of cage there was a marked difference in growth rate.

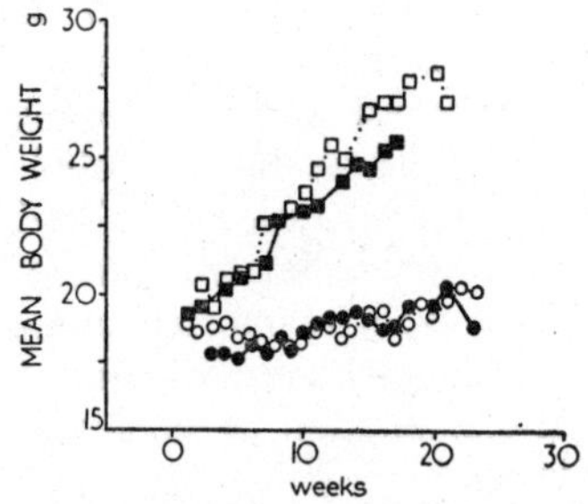

FIG. 20. Growth rate of female CBA mice and size of cage.
Standard cage containing four mice ■ MAXIMUM □ GAMMA
Small cage of half the standard volume containing two mice ● MAXIMUM ○ GAMMA
These mice were 8 weeks old at the start of irradiation.

Housing two mice in half the cage space almost stopped growth (as measured by body weight). It was also very noticeable that the saw-dust at the bottom of the cage had to be changed twice weekly in the small cages, although once weekly was sufficient in the large cages. The reasons for the differences between the two sorts of cage are not clear but the fact that the mice were not growing normally makes the observations on these animals of less value. They were used for tests of fertility, for blood counts and for obtaining weights of organs, and wherever the results are quoted they are listed separately from data obtained with mice housed in standard cages.

(iii) *Causes of Death and other Pathological Observations*

There was no visible difference between the mice in the different groups during the first nine months of the experiment. As body weight began to decrease in the MAXIMUM group, the hair became partially depigmented and sparser than in the other groups. Grossly visible lens opacities were not seen in the MAXIMUM group till after the end of the first year and their incidence rose rapidly about the time the death rate was rising rapidly. In the other groups similar though numerically fewer cataracts also occurred as a terminal event in mice which had lost a great deal of weight. Animals which had lost weight developed kyphosis and occasionally deformities of the sternum. Their bones were noticeably more fragile.

Every mouse was examined post-mortem for the cause of death with the exception of six which escaped at the weekly change of cage, seven where the body was destroyed in error and two fixed whole as specimens. Some of the bodies were so decomposed or eaten that only really gross lesions could have been detected. When calculating the percentage incidence of any lesion those animals have been excluded which were too decomposed for that particular lesion to have been detectable (as noted at the time of first examination). Each animal after exposure of abdominal and pleural viscera was fixed in corrosive sublimate-formalin and then preserved in dilute formalin. Each positive morbid anatomical finding was checked by at least one subsequent re-examination. Tissues were taken for histological examination as suggested by the naked eye changes, not as a routine.

Only in a minority of mice in any dose group was there an obvious anatomical cause of death; in the majority there was no apparent cause. Table 33 gives the incidence of the major categories of cause subdivided by dose and sex. No animal is entered under more than one heading. If a neoplasm was considered to be the primary cause of death the animal was entered in the category of 'killing tumours' even if the immediate cause was haemorrhage or intestinal obstruction. The definition of killing tumours is discussed subsequently (Chap. III, §2 (iv), p. 122).

After neoplasms, the commonest defined cause of death (six per cent) was intestinal obstruction, usually due to intussusception of the colon. If present this was usually complete, so that the intussusceptum often presented at the anus. The ileocaecal junction was always too bulky to enter the intussuscipiens so that the somewhat distended caecum was visible in the abdominal cavity. Deaths with intussusception of the colon occurred on the average at about the same time as deaths from all causes pooled together (Table 33). Obstruction at the ileocaecal junction with gross distension of the lower ileum by faecal material occurred less commonly but always at a younger age. No cause for either form of intestinal obstruction was identified (cf. Birrell, 1954).

Haemorrhage into the pleural or abdominal cavities from other than malignant lesions was the next most commonly identified cause of death (three per cent). Four pleural haemorrhages were probably due to pulmonary adenomata but in two cases this was

TABLE 33

Causes of death

	No. of mice	Local infection	Intus-susception of colon	Ileo-caecal obstruction	Haemor-rhage†	Killing tumours
Male						
MAXIMUM	49	0	2 (494)	1	1	8
Early death controls‡	48	0	1	2	1	8
MEDIUM	44	1	1	0	0	2
MINIMUM	47	0	1	1	0	1
GAMMA	45	0	6 (697)	1	1	4
CONTROL	45	1	0	0	0	3
Female						
MAXIMUM	50	1	1	0	0	13
Early death controls‡	22	0	0	0	0	15
MEDIUM	49	0	1	1	0	13
MINIMUM	49	0	3 (821)	1	0	12
GAMMA	49	0	3 (820)	3 (757)	0	12
CONTROL	39	1	0	0	0	8

Numbers in parenthesis are mean survival times in days.

† Excluding all cases where an underlying cause was found.

‡ 'Early death' controls are the combined mice from MEDIUM, MINIMUM, GAMMA and CONTROL groups which died between the start of the experiment and the 642nd day (inclusive), when the last mouse in the MAXIMUM groups died.

not proved. Abdominal haemorrhages in males were from hepatomata (two) and in females from ovarian and par-ovarian cysts (five) and angioma of the spleen (one). Haemorrhage into the gastro-intestinal tract possibly occurred often but was identified with certainty only occasionally because intestinal decomposition was so rapid. Such gastro-intestinal haemorrhages have been omitted altogether from Table 33. Blood counts were not done and deaths from anaemia were only recognized after severe haemorrhage or with leukaemia. No case of aplastic anaemia was recognized,

Localized infection (abscess) was found in six animals only, in the lungs in four, in the preputial glands in one and subcutaneously in one. Organisms were not seen in smears and culture was not done. Deaths from generalized infection would not have been detectable under the conditions of this experiment; bacteria in tissue sections were seen but rarely.

A small number of deaths were almost certainly associated with localized trauma to the abdomen, presumably caused either by bites or more likely by the claws of cage mates. A loop or loops of intestine would be found adherent to a damaged area of parietal peritoneum but there were no reliable signs of general peritonitis. In such animals autolysis seemed to be especially rapid and since this made diagnosis uncertain, these deaths have not been separately listed.

Some deaths were almost certainly associated with infarction of a large, usually pedunculated hepatoma in animals where the rest of the liver was smaller in size than the tumour, but as diagnosis here was also very uncertain these have also been omitted from Table 33.

Clear pleural effusions not assignable to any anatomical cause were found in two CONTROL, one MEDIUM and two MAXIMUM animals. No cardiovascular degeneration was observed with one exception (aneurysm of the left ventricle) and no definite lesions in the kidneys, except for pyelonephritis in three males. The glomeruli became relatively less cellular in aged mice. The papillary lesions and subsequent fibrosis described by Eschenbrenner and Miller (1954) were not seen although mites were commonly found on the hairs at death. Hydronephrosis was seen twice: it is found regularly in our mouse colony and seems to have little or no effect on the duration of life. Pneumonia and bronchiectasis were not seen, but as the mice aged, emphysema became pronounced. The central nervous system was examined rarely but deformities of the skull of the sort associated with pituitary tumours (Upton and Furth, 1953) were not seen.

Table 33 shows that there was no obvious effect of neutron irradiation on the incidence of any cause of death except possibly 'killing tumours', which will be discussed subsequently. The difference in incidence of intussusception of colon between CONTROL and GAMMA mice was statistically significant (for males only, $P < 0{\cdot}01$, for both sexes together, $P < 0{\cdot}001$, by Fisher's exact test). This presumably reflects some environmental difference other than irradiation (Chap. III, §2 (i), p. 100).

Tapeworms in the liver were seen in four mice. Multiple white nodules on the peritoneal surface of the caecum were seen in over half the male mice, never in females. They were more frequent in older mice which may account for the smaller incidence, twenty-five per cent, in the MAXIMUM group. These nodules were apparently identical with the para-caecal keratin cysts described by Burrows (1939).

Perhaps more important were the changes in the adrenal glands which were seen commonly in females and rarely in males. The external surface appeared to be studded with nodules varying from one to more than ten per gland, and marked out by their lighter, yellow colour from the browner, more translucent cortex around them. Histologically the glands showed a mixture of atrophy and 'nodular hyperplasia'. Much of the cortex consisted of cells very similar to those of brown fat, often separated from each other by 'septa' of spindle cells continuous with the superficial cortical spindle cells which replace the glomerulosa in aged mice. The recognizably cortical cells occurred in 'nodules' clearly defined in frozen sections by their fat content. These changes might have been regarded as merely senile but their macroscopic incidence in the females of the MEDIUM and MINIMUM groups (23 and 33 per cent respectively) was much greater than in the females of the GAMMA and CONTROL groups (4 and nil per cent). This was in fact the only difference found between the MINIMUM and GAMMA groups, but its relevance is obscure. The incidence in females of the MAXIMUM group was 40 per cent. Similar changes were the rule in CBA mice dying with leukaemia (Mole, 1955). It is possible that the nodules were the morphological expression of functional exhaustion of the adrenal glands.

(iv) *Incidence of Tumours*

When assessing the incidence of tumours difficulties arise. In this experiment mice were allowed to die naturally and post-mortem material is less useful for diagnosis than material obtained from the deliberately killed animal. This factor by itself would tend to underestimate tumour incidence, for in the absence of histological confirmation the diagnosis has not been recorded here, but the effect is not large nor likely to be important, except possibly when counting small tumours such as the pulmonary adenomata.

The second difficulty lies in choosing the appropriate control with which the comparison of an irradiated group is to be made. If an irradiated group with a shortened life-span is compared with a control group with a longer life-span, a decreased incidence of some tumours in the irradiated group could merely mean that the animals had not lived long enough for tumours to develop. Even if the incidence were the same in the two groups, it is not possible to be sure that irradiation decreased the induction period of the tumour without additional information about the rate of growth, and hence detectability, of the tumours. This additional information should ideally have been provided by separate control groups killed at predetermined times, or at random to match the duration of life of the irradiated group, but this was not done. Nevertheless, since the MAXIMUM group was the only one showing a really substantial shortening of life-span, it is perhaps legitimate to pool the data from the animals in the other groups dying during the same period of time, i.e. at the same age as the MAXIMUM group, and to use this pooled control group, called the early death controls (Table 33) as one basis for determining the effect of irradiation. Without pooling, the numbers are insufficient to make any useful comparison. Even so, it should be pointed out that the body weight of the MAXIMUM group was less than that of the pooled group of 'early death' controls, and that this nutritional difference, which it is impossible to control, may well be relevant.

The third difficulty lies in the low frequency of particular kinds of tumours. The strain of animal used, the CBA mouse, was chosen purposely for its natural longevity—which naturally entails a low incidence of 'killing tumours'. Even with 500 animals the numbers were many times less than the numbers required to establish, say, a doubling in incidence of a tumour normally occurring in one per cent of the population. And, as will be seen, to lump all 'tumours' together is not valid since the effect of chronic neutron irradiation appeared to depend on the particular kind of tumour under consideration.

Pulmonary Adenoma

Stewart (1953) and Orr (1947) have described the pathogenesis of this common mouse tumour, and their descriptions fit the examples seen in this experiment. The tumours were white sessile plaques on a pleural surface up to 2 mm in diameter or larger globular masses up to nearly 1 cm, rarely more than one per mouse and morphologically unlike pulmonary metastases of other tumours. No special effort was made to find all the adenomata, including the microscopic ones, as was done in the experiments of Henshaw *et al.* (1946) and Lorenz, Heston, Deringer and Eschenbrenner (1946), but every probable nodule seen with the unaided eye was taken for histological confirmation. In three of these cases no adenoma was seen in the sections and these have been excluded from Table 34. Just one unsuspected adenoma was found microscopically in the many lung sections taken for other reasons. The smaller adenomata and the edges of the larger specimens were histologically similar, being composed of closely crowded cells lying in irregular cords often with no space between them and with little visible stroma. The central areas of the larger tumours were often quite different showing a clear pattern of cubical or columnar cells lining narrow spaces and lying in a single row on both sides of a narrow core of stromal connective tissue. The transition to the peripheral pattern of growth was usually abrupt. There was no capsule.

These tumours rarely metastasize though they invade bronchi and may be disseminated widely through the lungs in this way. True intravenous growth was seen twice but no distant metastases were noted. Collapse of lung and distal infection from bronchiolar and bronchial obstruction might have been expected but was not recognized. In four mice death was apparently due to haemorrhage from a pulmonary adenoma but in two this was not proved. In one mouse, although the primary was not found, an adenoma had apparently ruptured into the pleural space causing a bilateral pleural effusion with metastatic deposits on pleural surfaces. With these exceptions the pulmonary adenomata appeared symptomless and without effect on the duration of life.

Table 34 gives the overall incidence of pulmonary adenomata in the different groups. There was no effect of irradiation except in

TABLE 34

Incidence of pulmonary adenoma

	Male		Female	
MAXIMUM	13/44†	30 %	8/43	19 %
'Early death' controls	8/43	19	0/14	nil
MEDIUM	9/42	21	6/45	13
MINIMUM	10/42	24	10/42	24
GAMMA	3/43	7	5/47	11
CONTROL	4/40	10	7/36	19

† In this and subsequent tables the number of animals with tumours is shown as a fraction of the number examined.

the male MAXIMUM group which had an excess of tumours significant at the five per cent level over the male GAMMA and CONTROL groups. The incidence in the MAXIMUM groups was not significantly greater than in the early death controls for either sex. It is not legitimate to combine the data for the sexes in view of the difference between the sexes in the relation between incidence and age (*vide infra*).

It is possible, however, to show the effect of irradiation in the female MAXIMUM group by considering the distribution of tumours with time of death. Normally, with a killing tumour, the probability of developing a tumour in a given time interval can be found from the ratio of the number of tumours appearing in this time-interval to the number of animals alive at the beginning of the time-interval. Pulmonary adenomata, however, are only rarely killing tumours so that the incidence must be determined by the proportion of animals dying in a given time interval which are found to have the tumour. Since in this experiment the numbers dying in any time interval were relatively small, the proportions fluctuate and the data for MEDIUM, MINIMUM and GAMMA groups have been combined (Figs. 21 and 22). The sexes are shown separately because there is a clear sex difference in the changes of tumour incidence with time.

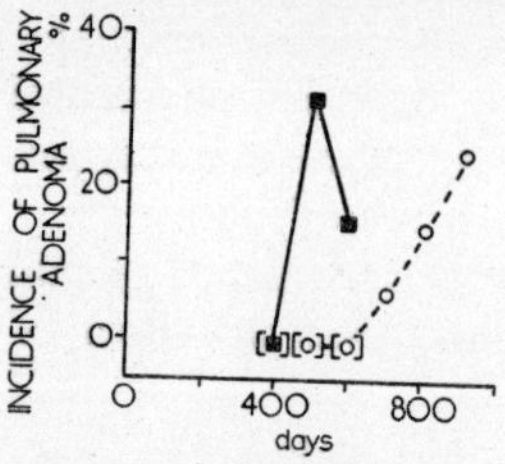

FIG. 21. Incidence of pulmonary adenoma (per cent) at autopsy of female CBA mice grouped according to survival time in 100-day intervals.

■ MAXIMUM

○ MEDIUM, MINIMUM and GAMMA together

Where there were less than twelve in a group the point has been bracketed

In all groups of females pulmonary adenomata were at first absent but, as the animals aged, appeared more frequently so that finally the overall incidence was between 10 and 25 per cent (Table 34). There was a clear effect of irradiation in the MAXIMUM group;

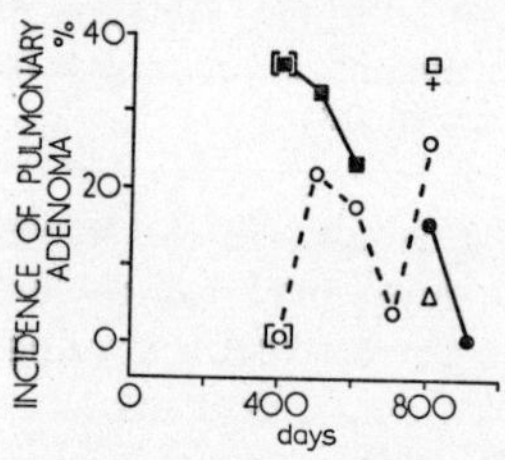

FIG. 22. Incidence of pulmonary adenoma (per cent) at autopsy of male CBA mice grouped according to survival time in 100-day intervals.

Symbols as in Fig. 21.

□ MEDIUM only 751–850 day group

\+ MINIMUM only 751–850 day group

△ GAMMA only 751–850 day group

● CONTROL only 751–850 day and 851–950 day groups

the induction time was shortened without any absolute increase in incidence.

In males, on the other hand, the pattern of tumour development with increasing age was different (Fig. 22). If anything, there was a decreasing liability to develop pulmonary adenomata with increasing age. This should mean either that in male CBA mice adenomata can regress or that, even if the tumours are not lethal, a male animal bearing an adenoma is liable to die earlier than one without. As it happens, the two apparently lethal pulmonary adenomata were the two early tumours in the CONTROL group. If adenoma do regress with increasing age the increased overall incidence in the MAXIMUM group could be due merely to the shorter life-span, as indeed suggested in Fig. 22 by the change in incidence with age up to the 750th day of the experiment. The incidence after this time was more than twice as great in the MEDIUM and MINIMUM groups as in the GAMMA or CONTROL groups and is possibly a real effect of low level chronic irradiation. This discussion illustrates some of the difficulties in deciding just how irradiation affects the incidence of a lesion. A simple comparison of overall frequencies in irradiated and control groups may be misleading.

Hepatoma

CBA mice normally have a high incidence of this tumour, an incidence which depends on age (Gorer, 1940) and on the composition of their food (Tannenbaum, 1953). The tumour is benign in the sense that it rarely metastasizes (Gorer, 1940), but may kill by causing abdominal haemorrhage or when a large tumour infarcts by torsion of its pedicle or otherwise. Often the hepatoma is larger than the rest of the liver and it is able to store glycogen and presumably carry on other functions of the normal liver. Hepatomata are often multiple. The tumours usually contain wide vascular channels and frequently show evidence of old haemorrhage and of necrosis. Histologically the tumour cells often, and the stroma occasionally, suggest an invasive habit of growth but in only one mouse (from the male MAXIMUM group) were multiple metastases certainly identified in the lungs. Sections of the periphery of a pulmonary adenoma sometimes suggested a hepatomatous origin.

TABLE 35

Incidence of hepatoma

	Male		Female	
MAXIMUM	20/44	45 %	16/44	36 %
'Early death' controls	28/45	62	5/16	31
MEDIUM	22/45	49	7/47	15
MINIMUM	20/45	44	11/47	23
GAMMA	9/43	21	6/48	13
CONTROL	14/43	33	3/36	8

The diagnosis of hepatoma in an individual mouse was less certain than the diagnosis of pulmonary adenoma because a thorough search within the substance of the liver was not made.

The overall incidence of hepatoma is given in Table 35. The incidence in females was always less than in males not only in the

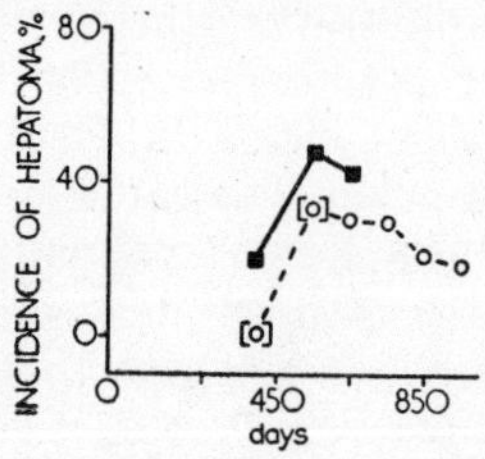

FIG. 23. Incidence of hepatoma (per cent) at autopsy of female CBA mice grouped according to survival time in 100-day intervals.

■ MAXIMUM

○ MEDIUM, MINIMUM and GAMMA together

Where there were less than twelve in a group the point has been bracketed.

controls (Gorer, 1940) but also in the irradiated groups, and the sex differences were significant for the MEDIUM, MINIMUM and CONTROL groups and the 'early death' controls. Differences statistically significant at the five per cent level were found between the male MAXIMUM and GAMMA groups and between the female MAXIMUM group and each of the female MEDIUM, GAMMA and CONTROL groups. There was no significant difference for either sex between the MAXIMUM group and the pooled 'early death' controls dying at the same age.

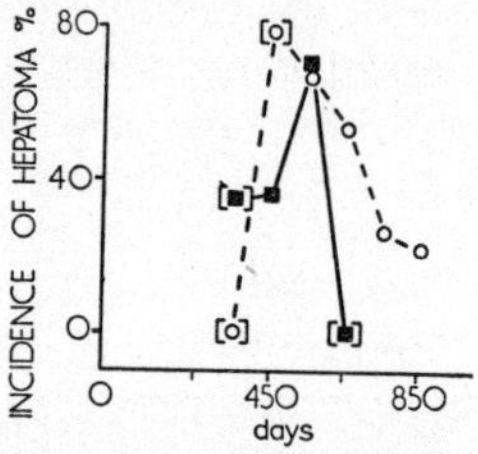

FIG. 24. Incidence of hepatoma (per cent) at autopsy of male CBA mice grouped according to survival time in 100-day intervals.
Symbols as in Fig. 23.

In Figs. 23 and 24 are plotted the probabilities of finding a hepatoma at autopsy in each 100-day period of the experiment. In both sexes, but more clearly seen in males (Fig. 24), there was a decreasing incidence of hepatoma as the animals aged. Examination of other CBA mice suggested that hepatomata first became visible between about nine months and one year of age when the frequency was already high. As with pulmonary adenomata one must assume either that hepatomata regress with ageing or that there is a link, not necessarily causal, between carrying a hepatoma and dying early. While it is true that the deaths which appeared to be the consequence of having a hepatoma, i.e. from haemorrhage and infarction, occurred amongst the early deaths, it seems likely from our other observations that hepatomata do regress with increasing age. The larger tumours were found in younger mice, and the haemorrhage and necrosis so often found histologically provide a probable mechanism for regression. If the natural history of hepatoma is indeed to decrease in size and frequency of occurrence with increasing age, then the comparison of overall incidence between the MAXIMUM and other groups is invalid for this tumour also. The data in Figs. 23 and 24 suggest that chronic neutron irradiation did not increase the incidence of hepatoma.

Tumours of Breast and Nasopharynx

These tumours are discussed under one heading because they were the only types of tumour with an apparently real increase in incidence in the MAXIMUM group, and therefore they provide the only evidence of carcinogenesis by chronic neutron irradiation obtained in this experiment.

Mammary tumours in CBA mice are normally very uncommon except when the mice are infected with the milk factor (Armstrong, 1948). Breeding tests in our stock failed to produce an appreciable number of such tumours showing that our CBA mice are free from the milk factor. The paucity of control material from unirradiated mice makes it impossible to make general statements about the natural history and morphology of the tumours in our colony.

The incidence of mammary tumours in the different groups is given in Table 36. The increase in the females of the MAXIMUM group over the combined MINIMUM, GAMMA and CONTROL females is statistically significant ($P = 0{\cdot}013$ by Fisher's exact test for 2×2 table). The occurrence in the MAXIMUM group of a mammary tumour in a male is perhaps of itself meaningful. The mean survival time of the MAXIMUM mice bearing mammary tumours was 419 days, 80 days shorter than the mean survival time for the whole group.

Histologically the tumours varied from well differentiated adenocarcinoma and adeno-acanthoma to mixed carcinoma-sarcoma with very few epithelial elements (cf. Eschenbrenner and Miller, 1954).

TABLE 36

Incidence of tumours of breast and of nasopharynx

	Mammary tumours		Tumours of nasopharynx	
	Male	Female	Male	Female
MAXIMUM	1/50	5/50	4/50	0/50
'Early death' controls	0/48	1/22	0/48	0/22
MEDIUM	0/49	0/49	0/49	1/49
MINIMUM	0/48	0/50	0/48	0/50
GAMMA	0/47	1/50	0/47	0/50
CONTROL	0/46	1/41	0/46	0/41

The nasopharyngeal tumours first presented as orbital swellings causing proptosis and metastases in the lungs. In three mice microscopic malignant deposits in the lungs led to re-examination of the head and the detection of orbital tumours with little externally to suggest their presence. After decalcification in versene the whole heads were sliced through and preparations made showing the whole width of the head. It was then clear that the growths had originated deeply and had spread upwards into the base of the skull, downwards to the epithelium of the roof of the mouth and laterally into the orbit. Although there was distortion by pressure, the growth did not cross far over the midline. Bones were eroded and the eyeball invaded but nerve trunks were not. Parts of the Harderian glands were recognizable surrounded by growth. Microscopically four of the five tumours were anaplastic carcinomata, one apparently a sarcoma.

The incidence of these nasopharyngeal tumours is given in Table 36. The mean survival time of the four males from the MAXIMUM group was 465 days. The greater incidence in the males of the MAXIMUM group as compared with the MINIMUM, GAMMA and CONTROL groups together, was statistically significant ($P = 0{\cdot}004$ by Fisher's exact test). It is interesting that all the tumours in the MAXIMUM group were in males but the occurrence of the fifth tumour in a female makes a real sex difference less likely. It may well be that the overall incidence of these tumours in this experiment has been underestimated, since those detected have been either big enough to cause an orbital swelling or have had pulmonary metastases. Smaller tumours without metastasis would not have been found by the methods employed: it seems difficult to obviate this except by serial sections of the head of each of the 500 mice.

Tumours of Female Reproductive Tract

In nearly all the females of the MEDIUM, MINIMUM, GAMMA and CONTROL groups one or both ovaries were brown in colour and up to 2–3 mm in diameter. A proportion examined histologically were senile or sometimes showed the tubular downgrowths described by Eschenbrenner and Miller (1954). In the majority of the MAXIMUM group, however, the ovaries were unpigmented and smaller. Simple ovarian cysts up to 1 cm in diameter were common except in the MAXIMUM group.

All ovaries of 4 mm and more in diameter were examined histologically and all were found to be neoplastic with one exception, an ovary consisting of tubular downgrowths of the surface epithelium of the type already mentioned. The neoplasms were either typical granulosa cell tumours, or histologically malignant growths. Intra-abdominal spread or pulmonary metastasis occurred in three carcinomata and one granulosa-cell tumour. Two presumed tumours (MEDIUM and GAMMA groups) were so destroyed by haemorrhage that no identifiable traces were found in sections and they are not included in Table 37.

TABLE 37

Incidence of tumours of the female reproductive organs

	Ovarian tumours granulosa cell	Ovarian tumours carcinoma (all types)	Other pelvic tumours
MAXIMUM	1	1	1 (2%)
'Early death' controls	0	0	4 (18%)
MEDIUM	1	4	1
MINIMUM	1	0	2
GAMMA	2	3	0
CONTROL	4	0	1

Two mice died from haemorrhage into par-ovarian cysts at about 500 days (one MAXIMUM, one GAMMA). There were four other large but solid pelvic tumours: one macroscopically, but not microscopically, a typical case of multiple uterine fibroids (CONTROL); two malignant vaginal tumours, one invading the rectum, the other with metastases in kidneys and liver (one MEDIUM, one MINIMUM); and a third vaginal tumour too decomposed for proper diagnosis but probably malignant (MINIMUM).

The incidence of these tumours is given in Table 37. The over-all incidence of tumours of the female reproductive system was about

10 per cent. and was less in the MAXIMUM group than in any other except the MINIMUM. The mean time of death of the animals with ovarian tumours was close to the mean survival time of the corresponding group, but the animals with large pelvic tumours died early. Thus the incidence of pelvic tumours in the 'early death' controls was greater than in the MAXIMUM group ($P = 0{\cdot}03$ by Fisher's exact test).

Tumours of Reticular Tissue

Typical common 'lymphoid leukaemia' of mice, with or without involvement of the thymus, is reasonably easy to diagnose. To classify all diffuse growths of the reticuloendothelial system into distinct categories is a much more difficult undertaking. Dunn (1954) has reviewed the subject and following her lead two other main categories will be recognized, reticulum-cell tumour type A and the mixed-cell, so-called Hodgkin's disease of mice (Dunn's reticulum cell neoplasm type B). The reticulum-cell tumours almost invariably presented with an enlarged liver, and usually with an enlarged spleen. Ascites and pleural effusion were common but mesenteric lymph-nodes were not usually enlarged. The degree of liver involvement was very variable and microscopically the cell-type was usually distinctive in some areas. Differentiation into spindle cells and vasoformative tissue occurred as described by Dunn, and in some sections histiocytoma (Gorer, 1946) would have been an appropriate description. These tumours occurred usually relatively early in life (Table 38).

The mixed-cell, so-called Hodgkin's disease of mice was found in older animals from 704 days on. There was always gross enlargement of the mesenteric lymph-nodes and often enlargement of the spleen. The liver was not enlarged. Microscopic diagnosis was hampered by the almost invariable autolysis and for the present purpose these lesions are considered not to be neoplastic.

One possible case of myeloid leukosis was found in a female mouse from the MEDIUM group but since the microscopic picture was not conclusive it has been excluded from Table 38. All other generalized leukoses not involving the thymus are included in the group of athymic leukoses: the majority were lymphocytic. The thymic leukoses occurred usually in younger mice (Table 38).

The over-all incidence of these lesions is given in Table 38. There were no differences between the irradiation groups, but female animals were affected several times more frequently than males, and the sex difference was more pronounced the earlier the age at which the animals died. If the MAXIMUM group is compared with the 'early death' controls, then for females the incidence of thymic

TABLE 38

Numbers and mean survival times of mice with tumours of reticular tissue

	Thymic leukosis	Athymic leukosis	Reticulum-cell tumour type A	Mixed-cell, so-called Hodgkin's disease	Angio-sarcoma
MAXIMUM	1	2	1	1	1
MEDIUM	2	2	2	1	2
MINIMUM	3	3	3	3	0
GAMMA	2	1	4	1	1
CONTROL	0	0	2	1	1
Male/female	0/8	2/6	4/8	2/5	0/5
Mean survival time in days (excluding MAXIMUM cases)	549	680	669	764	646

leukoses was 1/50 against 4/22 and of angiosarcoma 1/50 against 2/22. The former difference is suggestive ($P = 0{\cdot}03$ by Fisher's exact test). Other comparisons of MAXIMUM with 'early death' controls taking the sexes separately or together show small and non-significant differences only.

Vasoformative tumours both benign and malignant occurred, always in females. Angiosarcoma, locally invasive and metastasizing to the liver, appeared to originate near the pancreas (Table 38). Local angiomata of spleen and liver were histologically non-malignant but in one female of the MAXIMUM group appeared to be the source of a lethal abdominal haemorrhage.

Other Tumours

A variety of tumours were seen in such small numbers that little can usefully be said about them. There were two benign tubular adenomata of the kidney and six adrenal tumours. It is perhaps of interest, that two of the three adrenal tumours in the MAXIMUM group and one of two in the MEDIUM group were medullary and very similar to those described as phaeochromocytoma by Smith, Gardner, Li and Kaplan (1949) and found by them in X-irradiated mice. Two squamous cell carcinomata of the forestomach occurred late in life and one anaplastic gastric growth occurred early. Also occurring early were one carcinoma at the ileocaecal junction and one of two mediastinal new growths invading the lung, both in CONTROLS. Two sarcomata, one of the thigh and one at the base of the tail, were found in the MAXIMUM group; the animals bearing them died later than the group mean survival time. Females again preponderated by 3 to 1 taking all these tumours together.

The Simultaneous Occurrence of More than One Kind of Tumour

The frequency of occurrence in the same mouse of a pulmonary adenoma and a hepatoma, of either of these with a killing tumour, or of all three simultaneously, was consistent with the hypothesis that each tumour occurred independently of the others. The only suggestive link concerned adrenal neoplasms: of the three in females from the MAXIMUM group one was in a mouse with a granulosa-cell ovarian tumour and another in a mouse with a mammary tumour.

In their account of the results of chronic gamma irradiation Eschenbrenner and Miller (1954) emphasized the frequent association in LAF_1 mice of breast tumours and ovarian neoplasms (as defined by them), and implied that there was a causal relation, even though occasionally a breast tumour was found without a demonstrable ovarian neoplasm. The emphasis seems misplaced however, since the incidence of ovarian changes ranged from 60–100 per cent in their different groups so that from 60–100 per cent of mice bearing mammary tumours would have been expected to show the ovarian changes in the absence of any causal relation at all. There was certainly nothing in our neutron-irradiated mice to confirm the hypothesis that mammary tumours are in some way dependent on ovarian changes.

Killing by Tumours

It was not always easy to decide how important to an animal was the tumour it was found to carry. Tumours of breast and nasopharynx were always considered to be the cause of death. In addition, ovarian tumours with evidence of distant metastases, vaginal tumours, leukosis with or without thymic involvement, angiosarcomata and the carcinomata and sarcomata listed in a previous section were considered to be killing tumours. Reticulum-cell tumours were usually considered lethal except in three cases where the degree of involvement of the liver seemed insufficient. The mixed-cell, so-called mouse Hodgkin's disease was considered not to be lethal. In addition, a number of deaths were considered to be due to the effects of an otherwise benign neoplasm as indicated in previous sections, e.g. haemorrhage from ovarian and parovarian cysts, angioma of spleen and pulmonary adenomata. These are included in the group of 'killing tumours' in Tables 33 and 43. This selection is in some senses arbitrary but it is as true of the mouse as of man that autopsy, rather than demonstrating a cause of death, may merely reveal what it is possible to live with.

The mean survival time for the animals which died of killing tumours is given in Table 39 for each sex and group. It was always less than the mean survival time of the whole group and of the animals which were considered not to have died from neoplastic

TABLE 39

Mean survival times of mice with and without killing tumours

	Sub-group with killing tumours			Sub-group without killing tumours			Probability by *t*-test of difference in mean survival time of the sub-groups
	No. of mice	Survival time (days) Mean	S.E.	No. of mice	Survival time (days) Mean	S.E.	
Female							
MAXIMUM	13	473	26	37	524	17	< ·05
MEDIUM	13	633	48	36	803	14	< ·01
MINIMUM	12	709	49	37	833	12	< ·02
GAMMA	12	684	58	37†	819	16	< ·05
CONTROL	8	747	47	31†	845	24	not significant
Male							
MAXIMUM	8	441	30	41†	510	14	< ·05
MEDIUM	2	647	71	38	707	17	not significant
MINIMUM	1	543		46†	700	20	< ·001
GAMMA	4	581	29	41†	736	14	< ·001
CONTROL	3	463	37	43†	762	18	< ·001

† In each of these sub-groups it has been necessary when calculating the mean survival time to exclude one or two mice which were never autopsied (see Chap. III, § 2 (iii), p. 108). Their survival times were known and they are included in Table 23.

disease. The difference in mean survival time between the sub-groups killed by tumours and not so killed was statistically significant for each sex at each dose-level except in the female CONTROL group (and the male MEDIUM group where a statistical comparison is hardly justifiable). Shortening of life span by irradiation in the MAXIMUM tank was large in each sub-group of each sex but relatively greater in the sub-groups without killing tumours.

Separation into sub-groups did not reveal any significant shortening of life at lower levels of irradiation except in the comparison of males of the MEDIUM and MINIMUM tanks with the CONTROLS for deaths without killing tumours. Here the differences in mean survival time were possibly significant ($P < 0{\cdot}05$), but as noted earlier (Chap. III, §2 (i), p. 100), a fairer comparison is probably that with the GAMMA animals. The differences are then not statistically significant. It is unfortunate that the animals which have had to be omitted from Table 39 because they were not autopsied (and hence could not be assigned to either sub-group) were commonly animals dying early in the experiment. Nevertheless, even if all these animals are included in the sub-group without killing tumours, the conclusions are unaltered.

It has already been noted that some deaths were due to infarction of a large hepatoma and that large hepatomata were found in younger mice. The mean survival time of mice bearing large hepatomata, i.e. 1 cm and more in diameter, was usually about 100 days less than that of mice of the same group dying without killing tumours; but subtraction of the mice with large hepatomata from the sub-group dying without killing tumours did not alter appreciably the differences in mean survival time between the different irradiation levels. It has not proved possible to determine the exact importance of liver tumours as a cause of death in any group.

Interrelations of Body Weight, Tumour Incidence, Survival Time and Age at Start of Irradiation

It is often said that overweight individuals are liable to die earlier and even to have a higher incidence of tumours than those of average weight or less (Tannenbaum, 1953). The weight data already given (Figs. 18 and 19) show that a peak in body weight was reached between the 25th and 50th weeks of the experiment. For the purposes of this analysis male mice reaching 40 grammes and more and females reaching 35 grammes and more at some time in their lives, were considered to be overweight. These overweight mice occurred at random in the different cages (Table 40).

The incidence of killing tumours was not increased in overweight mice (Table 40). On the contrary in females of the GAMMA and CONTROL groups combined the incidence was less in the overweight than in the remainder (8 per cent and 28 per cent respectively, $P = 0{\cdot}01$ for difference by Fisher's exact test). The incidence of

TABLE 40

Incidence of killing tumours according to bodyweight

	Females				Males			
	Overweight†		Rest		Overweight†		Rest	
MAXIMUM	1/8	13%	12/42	29%	None	—	8/50	16%
MEDIUM	4/13	31	9/36	25	0/6	Nil	2/38	5
MINIMUM	3/11	27	9/38	24	0/11	Nil	1/38	3
GAMMA	2/18	11	10/32	31	1/10	10	3/37	8
CONTROL	0/8	Nil	8/33	24	0/9	Nil	3/38	8

† Overweight defined as weighing at some time in their lives 35 grammes for females, 40 grammes for males (see text).

pulmonary adenomata and hepatomata was the same in overweight as in other mice.

Further analysis suggested that mice entering the experiment underweight as compared with the average tended to have a higher incidence of killing tumours but it then became clear that such mice were often the mice of series III (Chap. I, §2, p. 4). When first put into the irradiation tanks these mice were some days younger than the other mice of series I and II. The data are given in Table 41 but the apparent increase in incidence of killing tumours with decreasing initial age cannot be considered as more than suggestive.

TABLE 41

Incidence of killing tumours in females according to age at start of experiment

Series	Age at start of experiment (weeks)	MAX.	MED.	MIN.	GAMMA	CONTROL
I	13½	5/20	4/19	3/20	3/19	4/15
II	13	3/20	6/20	5/20	6/20	3/15
III	12	5/10	3/10	4/9	3/10	1/9

The younger mice were also those whose mothers had taken longer to conceive, and some maternal effect could also be responsible. There was no significant correlation between age at start of the experiment and survival time.

The effect of overweight on mean survival time must be examined separately in mice with and without killing tumours since their mean survival times differed (Table 39). Unfortunately the number of killing tumours was few and a useful comparison can be made only in mice without killing tumours (Table 42). Male and female mice showed the same, unexpected pattern of results. Overweight mice in the MEDIUM and MINIMUM tanks lived longer than overweight mice in the GAMMA and CONTROL tanks. Mice which were not overweight, the 'rest', showed a progressive decrease in survival time with increase in dose rate of fast neutrons. Overweight mice lived longer than other mice when irradiated but less long when they were in the control groups. It is difficult to interpret these results which suggest that if an animal can respond to chronic irradiation by putting on weight, it will overcome the handicap of irradiation without incurring the additional handicap which overweight entails in the unirradiated.

In the sub-groups of mice not overweight, 'the rest', the shortening

TABLE 42

Effect of overweight on mean survival time of mice without killing tumours

	Female				Male			
	Overweight		Rest		Overweight		Rest	
	Mean	S.E.	Mean	S.E.	Mean	S.E.	Mean	S.E.
MAXIMUM	510	44	528	18	None		510	14
MEDIUM	831	16	795	17	752	16	662	24
MINIMUM	844	23	831	14	745	20	685	25
GAMMA	808	27	840	15	724	35	740	15
CONTROL	805	69	862	19	699	57	780	17

of life in the MEDIUM tank was statistically significant for each sex ($P < 0{\cdot}05$ for females, $< 0{\cdot}01$ for males in comparison with the corresponding GAMMA sub-group). The shortening of life of males in the MINIMUM subgroup was also statistically significant ($P < 0{\cdot}05$ in comparison with the malc GAMMA subgroup).

The Effect of Chronic Neutron Irradiation on the Incidence of Tumours

As already pointed out it is not always legitimate to compare the overall incidence of tumours in two groups of mice with differing mean survival times. In Table 43 are collected together the incidences of all the various tumours already discussed, in the MAXIMUM groups, in all the other groups pooled together and in the combined sub-groups which make up the 'early death' controls, *i.e.* all those mice dying by the 642nd day, the day the last animal in the MAXIMUM group died. It can be seen that the incidence in older mice was less than that in younger mice for six categories of tumour (Table 43).

The data for male mice are scanty and fail to show any effect of irradiation with fast neutrons at 6·4 rads weekly except for tumours of the nasopharynx. The apparent increase in pulmonary adenoma has already been discussed.

When the results for female mice in the MAXIMUM group and the group of 'early death' controls are compared, irradiation would seem to have caused a marked reduction in incidence of killing tumours (except mammary tumours). This is not a fair comparison however, once it is shown that the incidence of killing tumours normally decreases with age (see above). The 'early death' controls can then be used for comparisons only when a non-lethal lesion is being considered.

The overall incidence of killing tumours in females of the MAXIMUM

TABLE 43

Percentage incidence of tumours in MAXIMUM *groups compared with the incidence in the mice of the other groups combined*

	Female			Male		
	(a) EDC	(b) MAX.	(c) all	(a) EDC	(b) MAX.	(c) all
Pulmonary adenomata	nil	19	16	19	30	16
Hepatomata	31	36	15	62	45	37
Mammary tumours	5	10	1·1	nil	2	nil
Nasopharyngeal tumours	nil	nil	0·5	nil	8	nil
Ovarian tumours	nil	4	8			
Pelvic tumours	18	2	2			
Thymic leukoses	18	2	4	nil	nil	nil
Athymic leukoses	5	2	3	2	2	0·5
Reticulum-cell tumour	5	2	4	4	nil	2
Angiosarcomata	9	2	2	nil	nil	nil
Other killing tumours	9	2	2	4	2	1
Total incidence of killing tumours	68	26	24	17	16	6

(a) Early death controls, (c) all groups except MAXIMUM combined.

group was almost the same as in the females of all the other groups combined. Thus there was no evidence that chronic irradiation with fast neutrons was generally carcinogenic. Indeed, granted that the irradiation increased the incidence of one kind of tumour, mammary tumours, it would seem as if the irradiation must have decreased the incidence of other tumours in a compensatory fashion. The only suggestive evidence for this relates to killing ovarian tumours and unfortunately it is in the class of ovarian tumours that classification by pathological criteria differs most from classification by lethal effects. Only a quarter of the pathologically defined tumours listed in Table 37 were counted as killing tumours and the majority of the killing ovarian tumours killed by haemorrhage from pathologically benign or undiagnosed lesions.

Biologically, it is interesting that types of malignant disease which normally occur relatively early in life were not increased in frequency by irradiation in the MAXIMUM tank: here there is no question of the irradiated animals not living long enough for the lesions to develop. On the other hand, there was an apparently real increase in the MAXIMUM group in tumours of the breast and of the nasopharynx which, paradoxically, tend to occur late in life. Chronic neutron irradiation not only increased the incidence but must also have shortened the induction time of these two kinds of neoplasm.

3. EFFECTS OF LIMITED EXPOSURE

In the small cages already described (Chap. I, §7, p. 9) or in standard cages after they became empty by the death of the mice in them, additional batches of mice were put in the irradiation tanks and removed at intervals for blood counts, measurement of the weights of certain organs and histological examination of freshly fixed tissues, or for test of fertility.

(i) *Haematology*

Preliminary experiments showed that there were large differences of up to tenfold between the total white blood cell count in tail blood and in heart blood of normal CBA mice. The higher white count in tail blood was presumably associated with the slowing down of the blood flow in the blood vessels of the tail due to the inevitable cooling of the tail by the air surrounding it. This slowing of the blood flow would increase the accumulation of white cells in the thin layer of plasma lying immediately against the vascular endothelium and separating this from the mixed blood in the centre of the vessel lumen. Thus the white cell count in tail blood would depend on tail temperature and would be sensitive to changes of environmental temperature. All blood counts were therefore done on heart blood.

Heart blood was obtained in approximately 0·2 ml quantities by breaking the mouse's neck, pinning it out, opening the chest and inserting into the right ventricle a one-millilitre syringe with a wide bore needle but no piston. No anticoagulant was used and some expedition was required to collect successfully all the specimens required before the blood began to clot; sometimes one or other of these was lost. Red cell counting was done in Neubauer chambers, white cell counting in Fuchs-Rosenthal chambers (two chambers were always used and not less than 400 cells counted). Haemoglobin was estimated as oxyhaemoglobin in the M.R.C. grey-wedge photometer and expressed as per cent of N.P.L. standard. Blood smears were made on slides and stained by Leishman's stain; differential counts were made on 200 cells.

Table 44 gives the haemoglobin and total white blood cell count of CBA mice irradiated in the MAXIMUM and GAMMA tanks. There was no anaemia attributable to fast neutron irradiation and although there was a small decrease in the white count after six months' irradiation with fast neutrons in both males and females, neither decrease was statistically significant.

Total white cell counts were available for twelve litter-mate pairs

TABLE 44

Haematological findings during chronic irradiation by fast neutrons (6·4 rads weekly)

Duration of irradiation (weeks)		Sex	Mean haemoglobin per cent NPL standard		Mean total white blood cell count per mm³	
			MAX.	GAMMA	MAX.	GAMMA
3		M	105	102	2700	2100
5		M	108	109	1300	1600
9		M	—	103	—	1400
12		M	98	107	1200	2200
17		M	—	106	—	1600
26		M	97	97	2000	2000
30		M	95	96	1300	1900
40		M	97	—	2000	—
26–30	mean	M	95·9	96·7	1660	1950
(combined)	S.E.		±0·8	±1·4	±180	±230
26		F	97	99	800	1200

There were between 3 and 7 mice in each group at each time. The male mice irradiated for 3 to 12 weeks were in small cages (Chap III, § 2 (ii), p. 107), male mice irradiated for longer periods were in standard cages; the female mice were in small cages.

irradiated for 26 to 30 weeks. The white count of each irradiated mouse may be expressed as a per cent of its litter-mate control kept in the GAMMA tank: the two mice of a pair were always killed consecutively within a few minutes of each other and the counts similarly carried out together. The mean of these percentages was 81 per cent with a standard error of 5·9. Looked at in this way it is possible to conclude that there was a real reduction of 19 per cent in the total white cell count ($P < 0{\cdot}01$), but this small reduction was only demonstrable by comparing litter-mates. It is not possible to be certain that the reduction was due to the irradiation with fast neutrons since there were other unavoidable differences in the environment of the irradiated and control mice: the two groups lived in different cages in different tanks.

The lymphocyte count was approximately double the heterophil count in the GAMMA animals, and the proportions were hardly altered by fast neutron irradiation. Again there was no statistically significant difference except when the count in an irradiated mouse was expressed as a percent of its control litter mate. Then it appeared from examination of the twelve litter mate pairs irradiated for 26 to 30 weeks that the absolute lymphocyte count was decreased on an average to 78 per cent of the controls in the GAMMA tank by

TABLE 45

Body and organ weights (percentage of litter-mate controls, mean ± SE) in CBA mice irradiated with fast neutrons (6·4 *rads weekly*)

Duration of exposure (weeks)	Dose of fast neutrons (rads)	No. of litter-mate pairs	Body weight	Liver	Kidney	Spleen	Testis	Thymus
Males								
5	32	4	99±7	91±2	105±4	88±10	59±4	118±28
9	57	3	95±8	95±2	108±3	71±12	54±6	106±16
12	75	4	111±9	110±4	106±4	113±10	42±4	129±29
27	176	4	92±6	102±3	95±2	101±1	35±3	83±12
30	193	3	99±6	—	—	83±4	29±1	—
Females								
26	170	4	104±5	101±3	94±3	88±5	—	109±19

Each organ weight was expressed as a proportion of body weight and these proportions compared within each litter-mate pair, since the variability of the comparison was significantly less than when the absolute weights of these organs were compared. The loss in weight by the testis after 5 weeks was significant ($P < \cdot 01$). None of the other changes were statistically significant except the reduction in spleen weight after 30 weeks' irradiation which was not confirmed by later measurements (Table 46).

6·4 rads weekly of fast neutrons ($P < 0{\cdot}01$). The absolute neutrophil count was 95 per cent of the GAMMA controls.

It is notable that a level of chronic irradiation which shortened lifespan by one-third and produced a loss in weight after nine months' exposure, nevertheless caused only slight haematological changes after six months.

(ii) *Weights of Organs*

The weights of the freshly dissected testis, spleen, thymus, liver and kidney, were measured after continuous exposure of varying duration in the MAXIMUM and GAMMA tanks. For exposures of 3 to 12 weeks small cages were used, for longer exposures the standard cages. Litter-mate pairs were divided between the MAXIMUM and GAMMA tanks and a comparison made between each such pair. Mice were killed by breaking their necks and the weighing was done on a torsion balance. Since the heart was opened while it was still beating, all organs were weighed after exsanguination. The results are given in Table 45 and show that only one organ, the testis, consistently changed in weight.

Additional data on spleen and thymus weight are available from male mice (not litter-mates) kept for 40 weeks in the MAXIMUM and 48 weeks in the MEDIUM tanks and from CONTROLS of a similar age. The mean weights are given in Table 46 and show that at a time when

TABLE 46

Weight of spleen and thymus of male CBA mice after chronic irradiation by fast neutrons (6·4 *rads weekly*)

		Duration of exposure (weeks) 26–30	40	48
Spleen	MAXIMUM	54 ±1	59 ±5	
	MEDIUM	68 ±4		67±2
	GAMMA	60 ±2		
Thymus	MAXIMUM	18·5±0·7	16·5±0·8	
	MEDIUM	18 ±1·2		
	GAMMA	21 ±3		

Mean fresh weight in mg ± standard error.
All mice kept in standard cages.

the effect of fast neutron irradiation was beginning to show itself in a loss in body weight (Fig. 18) there was still no effect on the weight of spleen or thymus. The testis, on the other hand showed a progressive decrease in weight from much earlier (Table 45).

TABLE 47

Testis weight of CBA mice during recovery from a limited exposure to fast neutrons (57 rads in 9 weeks)

Interval from end of irradiation period (weeks)		4	12	18	24
Number of litter-mate pairs		3	3	4	2
Testis weight as per cent of litter-mate control	mean	48	68	84	89
	S.E.	4	4	4	4

These mice were never mated.

Further data on testis weight were obtained from CBA mice exposed for nine weeks in the MAXIMUM and GAMMA tanks, and then transferred to a radiation-free environment (Table 47). Examination at intervals thereafter showed that recovery of testis weight was a very slow process and was still incomplete five and a half months later. C57 Black mice and F_1 hybrids from A × CBA showed a similar incomplete recovery some months after removal from exposure to fast neutrons (Table 48).

TABLE 48

Testis weight of mice one year old after limited exposure to fast neutrons (6·4 rads weekly)

Mouse strain	No. of irradiated mice/ No. of controls	Dose of fast neutrons (rads)	Duration of exposure (weeks)	Radiation free interval thereafter (weeks)	Testis weight as % of control (mean)
C57 Black	4/3	104	17	25	71
ditto	3/3	128	22	20	68
F_1 (A × CBA)	4/10	78	13	31	93
ditto	3/10	176	30	14	72

These mice were tested periodically for fertility (Chap. III, §3 (iii), p. 136) their last mating being 4 weeks before the testes were weighed. They were all shown to be fertile during the two months before the testes were weighed.

(iii) *Male and Female Fertility*

The findings of Evans (1948, 1949) suggested that the gonads were among the tissues most sensitive to chronic irradiation by fast neutrons. The first experiment additional to the main survival experiment was an investigation of male fertility and the first results have already been briefly reported (Neary, Munson and Mole, 1953; the doses quoted in this paper have since been revised, Chap. II, §7 (i), p. 41).

Male Fertility

Method.—Male fertility was tested in a way similar to, but differing in detail from that used by Carter, Lyon and Phillips (1954). One male was placed with four females and left with them for four consecutive nights. Seventeen, twenty-one and twenty-four days later any visibly pregnant females were placed singly in other cages. From the 21st to the 25th days these cages were examined daily for litters and the number of young recorded. The young were then killed and the mothers returned to their original cage mates. Each cage of females was available for remating 28 days after the beginning of the previous mating period. Females were rarely used for more than three matings and never after they were six months old. With the exception of C57 Black females which gave unreliable results unless they were at least ten weeks old, female mice were first used for testing males when they were eight weeks old.

In the first series of irradiations, CBA males were tested for fertility before they were irradiated but experience showed that natural infertility was so uncommon that subsequently this pre-irradiation test was omitted. Marked males were randomly distributed between different cages in groups of four or five. The cages were then randomly allocated to different irradiation levels. The first series of animals were caged in the small cages which did not allow of normal growth (Chap. III, §2 (ii), p. 107). The results from these animals are recorded separately from animals housed in standard cages.

After a predetermined period in an experimental tank a cage of mice was removed for testing, as described, in a radiation-free room. At the end of the mating period the male mice were recaged together and usually returned to the tank for a further irradiation. This process was sometimes repeated several times, but never more often than at intervals of 28 days. After permanent removal from the experimental tanks the male mice were tested at intervals of four to five weeks to determine their recovery, if any. Over half the irradiated mice died accidentally from the toxic effects of chloroform vapour during the early recovery period: this is the reason for the marked drop in numbers tested (Table 50).

Results.—The results may be expressed in several ways: (i) the proportion of male mice found to be fertile as shown by fertilization of at least one female, however small the litter, (ii) the mean number of litters per male mouse tested (with or without the inclusion of apparently sterile as well as fertile mice in the denominator), (iii) the number of young produced per mouse tested or per fertile mouse

TABLE 49

Fertility of male CBA mice after various periods of fast neutron irradiation (6·4 rads weekly)

Group	Duration of irradiation (weeks)	Dose (rads)	No. of fertile mice/total no. tested: Irradiated continuously			Per cent fertile in all groups combined	Mean no. of litters		Mean litter size
			In small cages	In standard cages	Irradiated one day a week in standard cages		Per fertile mouse	Per mouse tested	
MAXIMUM	4	21–26	4/4	9/9	8/9	95	1·8	1·7	5·9
	5	33–34	5/8			63	1·3	0·8	5·5
	8	49–53	3/4	2/4	0/4	42	1·6	0·7	4·1
	9	55–59	1/8	6/14	5/9	29	1·4	0·5	3·7
	12	73–77	1/12			8	(1·0)	(0·1)	(3)
	13	83–84		0/10	0/9	nil			
MEDIUM	31	21		8/8		100	1·8	1·8	5·8
CONTROL		nil	15/16			94	1·9	1·8	6·3

or the mean litter size. This third index is less reliable than the other two because the female mice not uncommonly killed one or more of their litters, and inspection and recording of litter-size was made only once daily and at a varying time of day.

Table 49 shows how male fertility was impaired by irradiation in the MAXIMUM tank. There seemed to be no consistent differences in response between mice growing normally in standard cages or subnormally in small cages, or between mice irradiated continuously or given the same weekly dose but irradiated only on one day a week. There was no reduction in fertility in mice exposed in the MEDIUM tank for 31 weeks.

Recovery of fertility after terminating the irradiation began sooner after 9 weeks' than after 13 weeks' irradiation, and after this larger dose failed altogether in over half the animals (Table 50). The delay in recovery after the longer irradiation was shown not only in the time interval needed for return of fertility, but also by the smaller number of young produced at the first fertile mating. Fertility was tested at later time intervals, but the results are not shown in the table since male fertility began to decrease in unirradiated CBA mice more than 40 weeks old. Fig. 25 shows together the recovery of

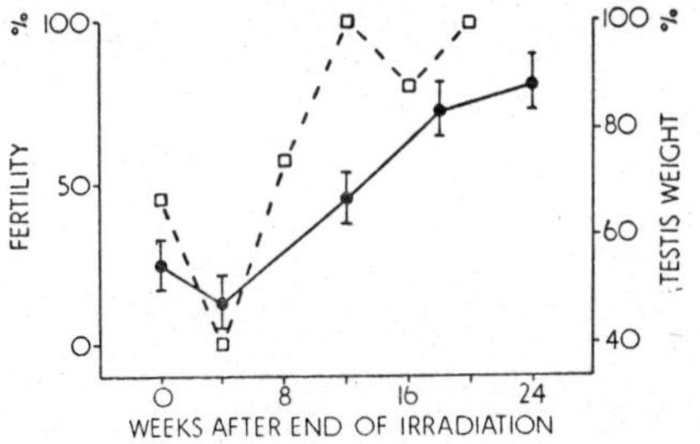

FIG. 25. Recovery of testis weight and of male fertility after nine weeks' irradiation of CBA mice by fast neutrons (6·4 rads weekly).

□ Fertility per cent (left-hand ordinate scale)

● Testis weight per cent of litter mate control (right-hand ordinate scale)

Zero fertility is plotted at the same level as 40 per cent testis weight because complete loss of sperm and spermatogenic elements entails a loss of no more than 60 per cent of the weight of the testis

fertility and of testis weight in separate batches of CBA mice irradiated for the same length of time, and it can be seen that testis weight was restored more slowly than fertility.

Male fertility after fast neutron irradiation was also examined in two other strains of mouse, C57 Black and F_1 from a cross between A and CBA. They were more resistant to irradiation than CBA mice, especially the F_1, but only small numbers were examined.

TABLE 50

Recovery of fertility in male CBA mice after a limited exposure to fast neutron irradiation

Duration of exposure (weeks) in MAXIMUM tank	Mean dose (rads)	No. fertile/No. tested Weeks after end of irradiation period 0	4	8	12	16	20	Mean litter si At first fertile mating test	At se fert mat te
9	57	11/23	0/23	8/14	5/5	4/5	5/5†	5·4	5·
13	83	0/19	0/19	2/19	3/19	7/18†	3/13	2·7	5·

These mice were all housed in standard cages throughout the irradiation period a as afterwards.

† Mice about 40 weeks old (see text).

The results on C57 Black mice (Table 51) show the same pattern of response as CBA mice (Table 50), but about twice as much radiation was required to produce the same effect. F_1 males on the other

TABLE 51

Irradiation with fast neutrons (6·4 *rads weekly*) *and fertility of male C57 black mice*

Duration of irradiation (weeks) in MAXIMUM tank	Accumulated dose (rads)	No. fertile/No. tested Weeks after end of irradiation period 0	4	8	12	16	20	Mean litter size of last two litters sired
13	73–83	5/13	2/5	4/5	4/5	—	4/5	5·7
17	97–104	3/8	0/4	2/4	3/4	1/4	4/4	5·1
22	128	0/4	0/3	1/3	3/3	2/3	—	4·8

hand were not even temporarily sterilized by 176 rads (Table 52). However, there did seem to be a reduction in litter size and in the mean number of litters per mouse while the mice were being irradiated, with some recovery on removal from irradiation (Table 52). The number tested was small but the mice in the different groups were litter-mates, and the males from (a) and (b) were tested with the same females alternately, so that the differences between the two groups were probably really due to the difference in the amount of radiation they received.

The C57 Black and F_1 mice of Tables 51 and 52 had their testes weighed at one year of age (Table 48). Comparison of these tables shows that in these two strains of mice also, fertility was normal

TABLE 52

Irradiation with fast neutrons (6·4 rads weekly) and fertility of male F_1 (A×CBA) mice

	(a)			(b)			(c)	
No. of mice in group	4			3			4	
No. of times sterile/total no. of matings during and after irradiation	1/28			2/21			1/8	
	Accumulated dose (rads)	Mean litter size at birth	Mean no. of litters per mouse per test	Accumulated dose (rads)	Mean litter size at birth	Mean no. of litters per mouse per test	Mean litter size at birth	Mean no. of litters per mouse per test
Tested after 13 weeks' irradiation	78	6·0	2·5	78	5·3	3·0		
Tested during next 17 weeks (4 tests each)	78	7·3	2·8	176	5·4	1·7		
During the following 9 weeks (2 tests each)	78	8·1	3·3	176	7·7	1·8	8·7	3·3

(a) irradiated for 13 weeks and then repeatedly tested while kept unirradiated.
(b) irradiated for 30 weeks, (tested at four-weekly intervals from 13 weeks on), and then tested four weeks and nine weeks after the end of the irradiation.
(c) control mice of the same age as (a) and (b) at the times of the corresponding tests.

or nearly normal at a time when testis weight was still only partially restored.

Female Fertility

Method.—Repeated tests of fertility during the course of irradiation are not practicable with females as they are with males, since either the females have to be kept unirradiated for a month at each test to avoid interference by radiation with intrauterine development, or the results are complicated by the effect of irradiation on the developing embryos. Female mice were irradiated continuously for predetermined periods and then removed from radiation altogether. The same day one male of the same strain was placed with each cage of females. The test male was changed at intervals of not longer than two months, sometimes much more frequently. The males used were from two to six months old during the time of mating: older males were not used in case their natural fertility was beginning to fail. The male was finally removed five months after the end of irradiation or when the females had reached the age when fertility had naturally disappeared, as determined on control unirradiated females. The cages were inspected regularly and each visibly pregnant female removed to a separate cage for littering. As soon as the litter was found, it was destroyed and the female returned to the cage from which it had been removed, from one to three days *post partum*. Each female was separately marked so that a record of individual performance was gradually accumulated. Occasionally pregnancies were overlooked, usually because the litter was very small, and littering then occurred in the mating cage. It was then not always possible to decide to which female the litter should be accredited.

Results.—The simplest method of recording the results was to determine the proportion of females which was absolutely sterile and the mean number of litters produced by a group of females irradiated together. Additional information was available on litter size and the interval between litters but these data are more liable to error, since litters were sometimes killed in whole or in part and since cages were not examined at weekends.

The results of irradiating CBA female mice in the MAXIMUM tank are given in Table 53. Irradiation is believed to prevent the development of Graafian follicles rather than to destroy mature follicles. Thus a dose of radiation less than that required to produce absolute sterility may allow one or two litters to be produced after the end of the irradiation but will lower the age at which an animal becomes permanently sterile. These changes were clearly shown by the mice given 108 rads in 17 weeks, and with the smaller dose of

TABLE 53

Fertility of female CBA mice after various periods of chronic irradiation by fast neutrons (6·4 *rads weekly*)

	Duration of irradiation (weeks)	Dose (rads)	Number fertile/number tested: Irradiated continuously (small cages)	Number fertile/number tested: Irradiated continuously (standard cages)	Number fertile/number tested: Irradiated on one day a week at 7 times the normal dose rate (standard cages)	Per cent fertility (combined data)	No. of litters per female tested (mean)	Mean size of first litter	Age at time of last littering (weeks)
MAXIMUM	13‡	83	4/4	9/9	8/8	100	2·6†	5·8	36†
	17	108	4/4	8/9	6/6	95	1·9	4·4	33
	22§	142	1/4	0/5	0/3	8	0·2	(3)	
	Age at mating (weeks)								
Controls	‡	Nil	8/8	11/11		100	4·6†	6·7	44†
	§	Nil	4/4	8/8		100	3·4†	4·8	48†

† Omitting the "small cage" animals which were not mated continuously.
‡ Mated for the first time at age 20–24 weeks.
§ Mated for the first time at age 29–32 weeks.

83 rads in 13 weeks the same pattern of response was seen. The number of litters produced was less than that expected from controls mated at the same age ($P < 0{\cdot}01$), and the age at which the last litter was produced was less ($P < 0{\cdot}01$). The size of the first litter in controls depended on maternal age and the reduction in size of the first litter by 83 rads was not statistically significant.

Comparison of males and females (Tables 49 and 53) suggests that, at 6·4 rads weekly, male fertility was more easily damaged than female. The sex difference was much too great to be accounted for by the difference in dose received by testis and ovary due to attenuation of neutrons within the mouse (Chap. I, §12, p. 26).

Data on other strains of mouse are given later (Chap. IV, §4, p. 169), and the comparison of the results on males and females for C57 Black mice (Table 51 and Fig. 41) and for F_1 mice (Table 52 and Fig. 40) shows that the relative sensitivity of the sexes was the opposite to that seen in CBA mice.

(iv) *Survival after Limited Exposures*

Various small groups of mice were exposed to chronic neutron irradiation in the MAXIMUM tank for limited periods, most of them for subsequent tests of fertility as already described. Many of these died accidental deaths as already mentioned (Chap. III, §3 (iii), p. 133) but all the others were kept till they died or developed a large visible tumour. The survival times of these female mice and the doses they received are set out in Table 54 and the effects of these limited exposures in shortening life seem clear. The data are plotted in Fig. 26 together with the survival times from the main continuous

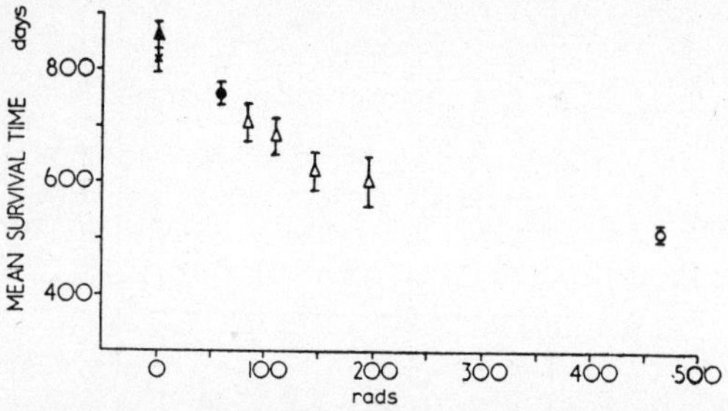

FIG. 26. Dose of fast neutrons (rads) and mean survival time (days) of female CBA mice after limited and continuous irradiation.

- o Continuous life-time irradiation at 6·4 rads weekly
- Δ Limited periods of irradiation at 6·4 rads weekly
- ● Continuous life-time irradiation at 0·54 rads weekly
- × Controls for continuous irradiation
- ▲ Controls for limited irradiation

TABLE 54

Limited exposure to chronic fast neutron irradiation and survival time (in days†) of female CBA mice‡

Dose (rads)	Duration of irradiation (weeks)	Daily irradiation No. of mice	Daily irradiation Mean survival time	Daily irradiation S.E.	Irradiation for one day weekly No. of mice	Irradiation for one day weekly Mean survival time	Irradiation for one day weekly S.E.	Combined No. of mice	Combined Mean survival time	Combined S.E.
83	13	8	767	40	8	639	45	16	703	33
108	17	9	668	44	6	697	51	15	680	32
143	22§	5	625	35	4	607	68	9	617	33
193	30§	5	599	45						
CONTROLS,	26§							18	862	24
MINIMUM and GAMMA								7	835	37

† A number of mice were killed because at the time they carried an obvious tumour. To the time at death of each of these has been added 100 days for the purpose of calculating the mean survival time of a group. The survival time of the controls was measured from the same age as the irradiated mice at the beginning of their exposure (8–9 weeks).

‡ The mice were those used for testing the effect of chronic irradiation on fertility (Chap. III, § 3,(iii), p. 138) with the exception of the MINIMUM and GAMMA group. They were housed in standard cages throughout.

§ Non-parous.

exposure experiment. The points lie on a smooth curve. Perhaps more interesting is the fact that the mean survival time for continuous exposure in the MEDIUM tank also lies on the same curve. It is tempting to take all this at its face value and deduce that 50 to 60 rads of fast neutrons whether given in a few months or spread out over a life-time would reduce the mean duration of life of female mice by 10 per cent. When such small effects are being looked for however, it is absolutely essential to have proper controls which are treated identically except for the factor under test, and these are lacking here: the number of litters born per mouse also varied systematically with the dose, thus introducing a further variable.

The overall incidence of killing tumours in the mice given limited irradiation by fast neutrons was 24 per cent, the same as in the CONTROL group of the main experiment. The latter were virgins however, and in the eighteen parous controls there was only one killing tumour (5 per cent). In the 31 parous irradiated mice there were 8 killing tumours, an increase which is suggestive, if not statistically significant ($P = 0{\cdot}07$ by Fisher's exact test). There were six adrenal tumours in the 45 irradiated mice and three examples of hepatoma metastasizing to the lungs. Neither of these was seen in the parous controls, and their incidence was much lower in the virgin females of the main experiment (Chap. III, §2 (iv), pp. 115, 121). These observations, if not conclusive of themselves, are in agreement with the suggestion that the carcinogenic effect of irradiation is more obvious after limited periods of irradiation than in animals given continuous irradiation till death (Mole, 1955).

(v) *Observations on Mice Bred in the Irradiation Field*

In a subsidiary experiment, a few males and females were caged together for a few weeks in the MAXIMUM tank. Several litters were reared and these mice had therefore been irradiated from conception. Their growth rate and maximum body weight were both definitely affected unlike mice which were 8 to 13 weeks old at the start of their irradiation (Fig. 27). The sex difference in body size was much reduced though still evident.

Some of these mice were killed at 11 and some at 42 weeks of age. Their haemoglobin levels and total white cell counts were in the normal range as judged by the data on normal mice in Table 44. The spleen and thymus formed the same proportion of body weight as in normal mice but the testes were atrophic.

The remaining mice were removed from irradiation at the age of 42 weeks. Their mean age at death was 545 days (males) and 522 days (females), so that their life span was shortened proportionately more than the mice irradiated from 90 days old. Among eight males there were two sarcomata, and two adenomata of the lung with intravascular invasion causing death from haemorrhage into the pleura; this incidence of malignant lesions was much higher than

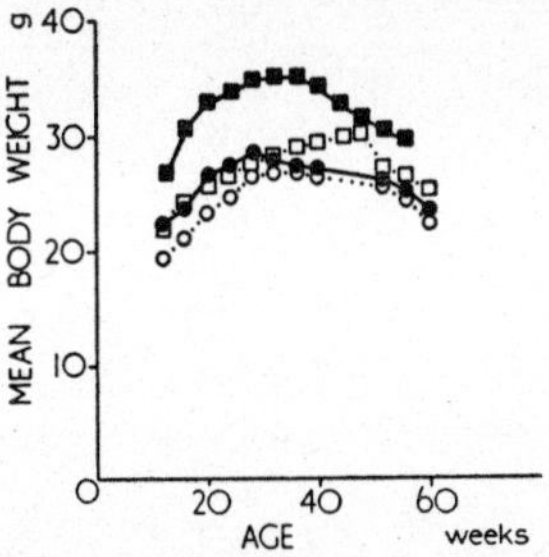

FIG. 27. Mean body weight (g) of CBA mice irradiated by fast neutrons from conception, and from maturity.

Each point is a four-week average. The weekly dose was 6·4 rads for all groups

■ Males, irradiated from maturity (mice of Fig. 18)
□ Males, irradiated from conception
● Females, irradiated from maturity (mice of Fig. 19)
○ Females, irradiated from conception

amongst the males of the main experiment. Among eleven females were found one malignant ovarian neoplasm and a tumour of the adrenal.

(vi) *Testis Weight after a Single Dose of Fast Neutrons*

During the second year of the experiment the mice being continuously irradiated were removed from the experimental tanks for one day each week (Chap. I, §4, p. 6). During this day the pile power was such that in the MAXIMUM tank the fast neutron dose was 6–8 rads in 24 hours, and advantage was taken of this to irradiate a separate series of male mice to test the effect on the weight of testis. Litter-mate pairs were allocated at random to control and irradiation groups a day or two before irradiation. The day the irradiation was completed, or the next day, each irradiated mouse was ear marked and again caged with its control litter-mate. Littermates were thus kept together in an identical environment and any differences found could confidently be ascribed to the irradiation. The weights of the two testes of the irradiated litter-mate were combined and expressed as a percentage of the corresponding control weight.

The effect of 6·5 rads of fast neutrons on the testis weight of mice of three different strains is shown in Fig. 30.* The general shape of

* See p. 161.

the curves is accounted for in the following way. The spermatogonia are the most radiosenstitive cells in the testis but they make up a small fraction only of the total mass of the testis. Loss of spermatogonia alone alters testis mass only slightly (cf. testis weight one week after irradiation). A reduction in the number of spermatogonia however entails a subsequent deficiency in the expected number of spermatogonial progeny. Since there is a continuous removal from the testis of the end-products of cell division, the spermatozoa, the main reduction in testis mass occurs some time after the loss of the spermatogonia themselves (cf. testis weight three weeks after radiation).

In the repair process the return of spermatogonia will not be reflected in an appreciable rise in testis weight. This will increase only towards the end of the successive cell divisions initiated by the spermatogonia.

4. DISCUSSION

The data given show that the plans originally made for this experiment were largely fulfilled. Biologically environment and general hygiene must have approached the optimum: there are few records of large groups of mice living to an average age of 800–900 days. Physically the weekly doses were kept reasonably constant and, though the average weekly doses were not as high as had originally been hoped for, they provided the information wanted. One dose level (in the MEDIUM tank) lay on the borderline between the definitely harmful and the apparently harmless, thus allowing an estimate of the 'tolerance' dose rate for mice. Another dose level (in the MAXIMUM tank) had a markedly damaging effect by some, but not all criteria, allowing an investigation of the relative sensitivities of different biological systems to chronic irradiation.

The general pattern of damage by chronic irradiation with fast neutrons was similar to that described for chronic irradiation of mice in general (Henshaw *et al.*, 1946, 1947; Lorenz *et al.*, 1947, 1954; Evans, 1948, 1949). There were many differences in detail from these earlier reports, some important, but nothing which could be picked out with certainty as peculiar to chronic neutron irradiation. Shortening of life span and damage to gonads were striking features in the earlier experiments on chronic gamma and fast neutron irradiation. The unfamiliar findings in the present experiment with CBA mice were the failure to find any general increase in tumour incidence in irradiated mice, the apparently greater radiosensitivity of the testis as compared with the ovary, and the relative radioresistance of the bone marrow.

Before these and other findings are considered in more detail, it is as well to point out one feature of chronic experiments such as these, which should not be overlooked when assessing the results. It is never possible to be sure that the sole difference between two groups given different experimental treatments is in fact due to the known difference in treatments. The longer an experiment runs the more likely it is that extraneous and undetected factors enter in, and in chronic experiments it is always harder than in acute experiments, and indeed often altogether impossible, to randomize things so as to allow for this. It would have been quite impracticable, for example, to have moved the tanks around periodically, or to have exchanged the fission and absorber layers in the different tanks so as to ensure that the apparently symmetrical arrangement of the animals and tanks did really entail uniformity of environment other than irradiation levels. A logical difficulty therefore underlies any deduction about effects of radiation based, as every such deduction must be, on a comparison between tanks.

When small differences are being investigated, and especially when the biological end-point is the result of the interaction of a large variety of processes, e.g. survival time, it is not only possible but indeed likely that the effects of irradiation will be magnified or obscured by undetected extraneous causes. The difference in mean survival time between CONTROL and GAMMA tanks is a case in point. We can be sure that this was not due to the difference in irradiation levels, for if so there should have been a much greater difference than was in fact observed between the mean survival times in the GAMMA and MINIMUM tanks. It is actually a fortunate circumstance that the weekly dose in the MINIMUM tank was so low. If it had been as high as originally planned and the mean survival time correspondingly shortened, the difference in mean survival time between the GAMMA and CONTROL tanks might have been taken to be due to the small neutron dose in the GAMMA tank (Table 19) and this would have given a correspondingly exaggerated impression of the killing power of fast neutrons, in confirmation of the suggestions that the r.b.e. for killing effect was really very large (see Chap. I, §3, p. 5).

The experiment of Lorenz *et al.* (1954) also illustrates the point under discussion. The mean survival time of mice given 0·1 r daily of gamma radiation was greater than that of unirradiated control mice ($P = 0{\cdot}1$). It seems to us improbable that low level irradiation should prolong life, and the description of the experimental arrangement shows that the mice given 0·1 r daily were kept in a different room from the controls and the other mice given higher daily doses. It seems to us far more likely that it was this environmental difference which was responsible for the difference in mean survival times. And not only this. The incidence of ovarian tumours was greater in the group given 0·1 r daily than in the unirradiated controls, an experimental result which has often been quoted to show the harmful effects of this level of chronic irradiation. But if ovarian tumours (as defined by these authors) become common in really old mice (as was seen in our CBA mice), the difference between the mice given 0·1 r daily and the control mice in the shape of the mortality curves, and hence in the proportion surviving to old age (Lorenz *et al.*, 1954), may of itself be sufficient to explain the difference in incidence of ovarian tumours, which may thus also be a consequence of an environmental difference between the two groups of mice other than irradiation.

Great pains were taken, as described in Chap. I, to keep the environment as similar as possible in all tanks but the mean survival times in the GAMMA and CONTROL tanks (Table 23) and the difference in incidence of intestinal obstruction (Table 33) show that we did not completely succeed. Nevertheless the uncontrolled differences between the GAMMA and the other irradiated tanks are likely to have been much less than between the GAMMA and the CONTROL tanks because of the general experimental layout (Chap. I, §1, p. 2, §4, p. 6, §6, p. 8, Figs. 1 and 3), and we do not believe that they invalidate any of our deductions. The similarity of the results in the GAMMA and MINIMUM tanks in almost every respect is evidence in support of this belief.

Tumour Incidence and Causes of Death

The incidence of tumours and of discoverable causes of death are obviously closely related and will be discussed together. It is clear first of all that, if a neoplasm takes a certain time to develop, a dose level of chronic irradiation which kills before that time has elapsed may reduce the incidence of the neoplasm. This was the explanation offered by Henshaw *et al.* (1946) for the pronounced reduction in lymphoma incidence in C58 mice when this high lymphoma strain was irradiated with fast neutrons or gamma rays. In the present experiment the mean survival time in the MAXIMUM tank was less than the mean time to death for any variety of tumour of the reticuloendothelial system in the other groups (Table 38), and this may help to account for the absence of any increase in frequency of these lesions in the MAXIMUM group.

A high incidence of lymphoma in chronically irradiated mice has been reported by others. Female LAF_1 mice irradiated with 8·8 r daily of gamma radiation showed a lymphoma incidence of over 60 per cent compared with under 50 per cent in controls (Lorenz *et al.*, 1954). CF_1 mice irradiated with fast neutrons (Henshaw *et al.*, 1946) are stated to have shown a 50 per cent incidence of lymphoma compared with 10 per cent in the controls. No details were given, and a much higher incidence in untreated CF_1 mice was reported by Finkel, Lisco and Brues (1954). For ABC mice (Henshaw *et al.*, 1946) details are not given but it is stated that leukaemia incidence was not greatly altered by chronic irradiation with fast neutrons. In general it seems to be true that, where lymphoma incidence was high, unexplained deaths were low in frequency and vice versa, both in irradiated and control groups, but that an increase in the frequency of lymphoma has not been a striking effect of chronic irradiation except possibly in the CF_1 mice mentioned above.

However, the conditions of irradiation may be of overriding importance. CBA mice, which did not show any increase in leukaemia as a result of continuous irradiation in the MAXIMUM tank, nevertheless showed a striking increase when given a limited period of daily X-irradiation (Mole, 1955, 1956). Further work is needed to decide whether this difference is due to a real difference in the leukaemogenic efficiency of different kinds of radiation or to such technical factors as the duration of the irradiation period or the proportion of the day which is radiation-free.

The CBA mice given continuous irradiation till they died lost a great deal of weight over a long period. It is well known that calorie restriction may reduce the incidence of detectable tumours, and the leukaemogenic effect of the fast neutrons may thus have been masked by their other actions.

The genetic composition of the mouse strain used would also be expected to be relevant. Henshaw *et al.* (1946) commenting on their results with C58 mice state that a high natural incidence of leukaemia did not ensure a high leukaemogenic response to radiation. The relatively small increase in incidence in LAF_1 mice (Lorenz *et al.* 1954) bears this out.

The differential effect of chronic neutron irradiation in our experiment on two main classes of tumours has already been noted. Tumours which normally occurred in middle age were not increased in frequency, tumours which normally occurred rarely and late in life were increased in frequency and occurred earlier. No similar finding seems to have been noted by others. The results could indicate merely a differential sensitivity of the two classes of tumours to nutritional insufficiency of the host. There might also be some difference in the radiosensitivity of the tumour induction process in the two classes of tumours.

Detailed data of the incidence of a variety of tumours were given earlier, and it was pointed out that it was sometimes necessary to consider the change in incidence with age before assessing the effect of irradiation. This was the case with pulmonary adenomata in female CBA mice, where the overall incidence at death after 6·4 rads weekly was the same as in controls, but where there was a clear effect of irradiation in shortening the induction period with a definite increase in incidence in irradiated mice compared with controls dying at the same age. A sex difference in the relation between incidence and age was also noted: in male CBA mice the incidence decreased with age as in LAF_1 mice (Lorenz *et al.* 1954).

A more searching technique for locating lung tumours was used by Henshaw *et al.* (1946) and Lorenz *et al.* (1946). Also the control mice (of a high lung tumour strain, strain A), were killed at the same time (9–12 months of age) as the irradiated, so obviating interpretative difficulties depending on age differences. In one experiment fast neutrons at 1·15 n daily (14 rads weekly) did not increase the incidence of lung tumours, in both experiments gamma irradiation at between 8 and 9 r daily did, by about 60 per cent. The only effect of the fast neutrons was to increase markedly the number of tumours carried by each tumour-bearing animal. In CBA mice this effect was not noted.

These observations, that chronic irradiation failed to increase the incidence of lymphomas and lung tumours by as much as two-fold in strains of mice with a high natural incidence, may not mean that the carcinogenic action of such irradiation is weak. An alternative possibility is that the high natural incidence in these strains is a consequence of some event(s) occurring early in life and uninfluenced by subsequent irradiation. If this be so, strains with a high natural incidence of tumours are to be avoided in experiments on carcinogenesis by irradiation for any additional neoplasms caused by the irradiation will then appear as a small increase over a high baseline frequency. The same number of irradiation tumours added to a low control frequency might provide a much more striking demonstration of carcinogenic potency.

Thus the CBA mice used in our neutron experiment and the LAF_1 mice used by Lorenz *et al.* (1954) in their gamma ray experiment were strains with a very low natural incidence of mammary tumours, so that the occurrence of a small number of mammary tumours in the irradiated groups was important. An incidence of 10 per cent may represent a fivefold increase and demonstrate a real carcinogenic effect. In both these experiments chronic irradiation shortened the induction time of mammary tumours as well as increasing their frequency.

When allowance has been made for all possible causes of death, it still remains true in our experiment that a large proportion of mice from all groups died without assignable cause. This is also true of a not inconsiderable proportion of human post mortems and the mouse pathologist is additionally handicapped by the absence of clinical notes and investigations, by the rapidity with which mouse tissues may autolyse, and by the cannibalistic habits of the dead mouse's cage mates. The frequency of unexplained deaths in irradiated mice was not higher than in the unirradiated.

Other Effects

Some manipulation of the observed data was needed in order to show that any of the differences from controls produced by 0·54 rads weekly were statistically significant (Chap. III, §2 (i) and (iv), pp. 97 and 126). Nevertheless, all the differences were in the same direction suggesting that this weekly dose rate might have been harmful. Survival time was shortened in both male and female mice, especially if later deaths were considered (Chap. III, §2 (i), p. 97) or overweight mice excluded (Chap. III, §2 (iv), p. 126 and there was also a possible increase in pulmonary adenoma in aged males. There was a slightly earlier fall in weight in males and a slightly faster rate of weight loss in females than in the MINIMUM or GAMMA tanks. The incidence of microscopically abnormal adrenal glands in females was greater than in the GAMMA or CONTROL females. The increase in incidence of abnormal adrenal glands and of pulmonary adenomata was shared by the corresponding MINIMUM group and no secure conclusions are possible.

However, to search for specific morphological consequences of chronic irradiation and compare their frequency in groups irradiated at different levels may not really be an appropriate technique for disclosing the harmful effect of chronic irradiation. Death may well result from the combination of a number of subliminal functional deficiencies, each not significantly greater than in controls but together summating or even potentiating their effects. In these circumstances the overall effect is likely to be a more sensitive index of harm than any individual item. The survival time is often taken as such a measure of overall effect and a fairly exhaustive analysis of survival times in whole groups and in variously defined sub-groups was made above. The shape of the survival curves suggested that each was perhaps composed of two components, one accounting for the earlier deaths which tended to straggle out in time, the other for the later deaths which tended to occur much closer together (Figs. 14 and 15). This analysis agreed fairly well with the independent pathological division between the sub-groups dying with and without killing tumours (Table 39). Animals dying without killing tumours were usually those dying without a well-defined cause and, if this is taken as the definition of dying from old age, the hypothesis that chronic irradiation causes premature ageing may perhaps be thought to have some pathological support.

Lorenz *et al.* (1947) observed that daily gamma irradiation at doses so low that the effect on life span was equivocal or slight nevertheless increased bodyweight, and this was subsequently confirmed in a repeat experiment (Lorenz and Jacobson, 1949). In our CBA mice irradiated with fast neutrons there was no such effect, though it was also shown by female CF_1 mice irradiated with 0·115 n daily (Henshaw *et al.* 1946).

We found that a dose rate of fast neutrons (6·4 rads weekly) which produced little alteration in the number of either granular leucocytes or lymphocytes in the blood, was nevertheless sufficient to shorten life very considerably. This confirms the findings of earlier workers with mice (Lorenz *et al.*, 1947, with gamma radiation, Henshaw *et al.*, 1946, with gamma radiation and fast neutrons). Dose rates sufficient to produce a substantial decrease in the white blood count in mice shortened life by more than 50 per cent (Henshaw *et al.*, 1946; Evans, 1948; unpublished observations of our own). The generally accepted view that blood counts are of value as a protective measure to man occupationally exposed to radiation has been criticized on other grounds (Mole, 1954).

Importance of Recovery

In a second experiment referred to briefly later (Chap. IV, §1, p. 156), in which mice were given a higher weekly dose, 16 rads of fast neutrons, there was a real decrease in total white count to less than half that of litter-mate controls. The main fall in white count occurred during the first five weeks and thereafter the rate of fall progressively diminished (Fig. 42). The pattern of change was that to be expected from a balance between continued damage and continued repair (Mole, 1954). This would explain why at the lower dose rate of 6·4 rads weekly there was so little change in the white count: at this smaller dose rate repair was able to keep pace with the lesser rate of damage. If this general view is correct, it might appear at first sight to confirm the method of basing the maximum permissible dose rate on an absence of changes in the white cell count of the peripheral blood, for this would indicate that the rate of radiation damage was within the capacity of the body to repair itself. The possible dangers of keeping a repair process in the bone marrow at full or even half stretch would then need consideration, e.g. on the somatic mutation theory of carcinogenesis, any increase in the number of cell divisions must increase the risk of malignant disease.

The lymphocyte count was depressed earlier and to a proportionally greater extent than the heterophil count during exposure to 16 rads weekly (unpublished observations). The same tendency was observed at the lower weekly dose of 6·4 rads and it may be concluded that in the mouse, just as for gamma radiation (Lorenz *et al.*, 1954) so also for fast neutrons, lymphocytes are more sensitive than heterophils as an index of chronic irradiation.

A preliminary report on damage to the gonads by chronic irradiation with fast neutrons has already been published (Neary, Munson and Mole, 1953). The gonads of CBA mice were found to be more sensitive than the bone marrow or lymph nodes. Evans (1948) also found that sterilization of male mice by fast neutrons occurred well before the maximum change in the white blood count, and Deringer, Heston and Lorenz (1954) found that female LAF_1 mice were sterilized by 4·4 r daily of gamma radiation at a time when the blood count had hardly altered (Lorenz *et al.*, 1954). The greater sensitivity of the gonads as compared with the bone marrow is therefore not peculiar to CBA mice or fast neutron irradiation.

The relative sensitivities of the gonads of the two sexes has varied from experiment to experiment in a way which cannot be accounted for by differences in dose distribution within the mouse and thus in the actual dose received by the testis or ovary (Chap. I, §12, p. 26). In Evans's Swiss mice and our CBA mice irradiated with fast neutrons, the males were more easily sterilized than females. On the other hand females were more sensitive than males in the experiments of Deringer *et al.* (1954) with gamma irradiation of LAF_1 mice, and in our experiments with fast neutron irradiation of F_1 hybrid and C57 Black mice (cf. Table 52 with Fig. 40 and Table 51 with Fig. 41). Besides differences between mouse strains in intrinsic radiosensitivity of the ovaries to fast neutrons and gamma radiation (Chap. IV, §4, p. 169), there are also differences between strains of mice in the capacity of the testis to recover after irradiation. The lower the daily dose the better the chance the male has to repair radiation damage and to appear more resistant than the female.

Any attempt to determine experimentally the most sensitive criterion of chronic radiation damage must take into account the capacity to recover in the face of continued irradiation. This is also directly relevant to the determination of relative biological efficiencies as shown subsequently. Even if initial damage were the same for all mouse strains (or all species of mammals), which is conceivably true if damage depends purely on the interaction of physical or chemical products of radiation with molecules of the same general structure in all mouse strains (or mammals), e.g nucleic acid, there is no *a priori* reason why the rate of biological recovery should be the same. The rate of recovery must depend on many of the metabolic and structural features which distinguish strains and species. Thus it is to be expected that the most sensitive criterion of chronic radiation damage will differ according to the particular species examined, as was made clear by the comparative results of Lorenz *et al.* (1954) in guinea-pigs, rabbits and mice.

In addition, there are clearly pitfalls in comparing the relative sensitivity of different organs when the radiation damage is revealed by tests of arbitrary design which may differ markedly in the intensity with which they test functional capacity, and hence in the efficiency with which they reveal small functional deficiencies. The methods used by all those cited earlier differed in many details even when the same function, fertility, was being examined. Fertility testing of males and females is inevitably different, e.g. males are potentially fertile at any time, females only periodically. More important still is the impossibility of comparing an organ able to recover from radiation damage, the testis, with one in which damage may be irreparable, the ovary. It is therefore illegitimate to conclude from a comparison of the results already discussed that there is any general difference in the relative sensitivity of the gonads of the two sexes to chronic neutron and gamma radiation, and it is impossible also, for the same reasons, to determine, in any absolute sense, the relative radiosensitivities of the different tissues of the body.

Nevertheless, from the human, toxicological point of view it is of great importance to know what part of the body is most easily damaged by chronic irradiation. Direct evidence from human experience is very scanty, and what there is suggests that testicular atrophy preceded serious bone marrow damage by a long interval (Mole, 1954). Not only the experiments on mice already discussed but also the effects of daily irradiation at 1 r daily and less in dogs (Casarett and Hursh, 1956) suggest that of all the functions so far examined the reproductive function is the most easily damaged by chronic irradiation. Guinea pigs are an exception (Lorenz *et al.*, 1954), and when applying the results of animal experiments to man it is necessary to use some criterion of selection. Lorenz (1954) suggested that man should be considered as sensitive as that species of animal found experimentally to be the most sensitive. Lorenz's criterion may well be the safest but it should be pointed out that its application may mislead. The wider the range of species examined the more sensitive is the most sensitive likely to be. Yet there seems no intrinsic reason to believe that man is necessarily at the lower limit of the mammalian range of radiosensitivities for all functions of importance. More work and a strict application of Lorenz's criterion might easily lead to a wrong idea of the relative radio-sensitivities of different functions in man. In fact, it is only human experience that can give us certainty in any case. And lastly there still remains the peculiarly human problem of values: which is the most harmful, cataract of the eye, damage to the gonads or an increased liability to cancer?

One point which should perhaps be stressed is the unexpectedly large effect on life span of a limited exposure to daily irradiation. For daily X ray exposures at relatively high dose rates this has already been reported (Mole, 1955) but Fig. 26 suggests that for fast neutrons also it is the first few months of a chronic exposure which largely determine the outcome. Subsequent radiation becomes less effective as the irradiation continues.

5. SUMMARY

(1) Four exposure areas, each adequate for irradiating continuously one hundred mice at a time, gave weekly doses of fast neutrons ranging from 0·08 to 6·4 rads. The gamma contamination was reduced to less than 1 r weekly except in the tank with the highest neutron dose. The irradiation was almost continuous: on the average 26 hours a week were free from irradiation during the two and a half years of the experiment.

(2) The mean survival times of CBA mice in the control groups were 743 days for males and 818 days for females, measured from the start of the experiment when the mice averaged 90 days of age.

(3) The mean survival time was decreased by a third by a weekly dose of 6·4 rads of fast neutrons. The significance of the small decrease in mean survival time at 0·54 rads weekly depended on the method of analysis.

(4) Two hypotheses accounting for the distribution of deaths with time were critically considered: (a) radiation acts independently of other causes of death and superimposes an excess mortality upon the natural mortality, (b) radiation interacts with natural causes of death so as to make them effective earlier or prematurely.

(5) The majority of the mice, both irradiated and controls, died without the cause of death being discovered post-mortem. There were a small proportion of deaths from intestinal obstruction, commonly an intussusception of the colon, and a larger proportion due to killing tumours. A full analysis of the post mortem findings is given.

(6) The incidence of some 'killing' tumours decreased as mice became aged. Obesity (as judged by a comparison of body weight with the average) did not predispose to earlier death.

(7) Mammary tumours and malignant tumours of the nasopharynx were increased in incidence by 6.4 rads weekly of fast neutrons. The incidence of other malignant tumours was unchanged or decreased.

(8) After allowing for change in incidence with age, pulmonary adenomata increased in frequency and had their induction time shortened in female mice given 6·4 rads weekly. The effect in males was less clear.

(9) There was an abrupt onset of weight loss after about nine months at 6·4 rads weekly but no evidence at any dose rate of a tendency to increase in weight.

(10) No light was thrown on the cause of death after irradiation for life by examination of tissues after a few weeks or months of irradiation.

(11) The white blood cell count was of no value in predicting radiation damage. The thymus and spleen were also insensitive indicators of chronic radiation damage. Blood lymphocytes were more sensitive than heterophils to chronic neutron irradiation.

(12) By far the earliest change detected was damage to the gonads. The relative sensitivities of testis and ovary varied with the strain of mouse examined. Gonadal damage was approximately the same whether the weekly dose was given in one day or seven. The weight of the testis was a more sensitive indication of radiation damage than fertility in the conditions used.

(13) The problem of determining the relative radiosensitivities of different organs is critically discussed. No simple extrapolation to man is possible.

(14) An exposure to chronic irradiation limited to a few weeks or months resulted in a shortening of the life span. Continued irradiation till death over-estimated the amount of radiation required to shorten the life span by a given amount.

REFERENCES

Armstrong, E. C., *Brit. J. Cancer*, 1948, **2,** 59.
Birrell, J., *J. Path. Bact.*, 1954, **67,** 617.
Burrows, H., *J. Path. Bact.*, 1939, **49,** 260.
Carter, T. C., Lyon, M. F., and Phillips, R. J. S., *Brit. J. Radiol.*, 1954, **27,** 418.
Casarett, G. W., and Hursh, J. B., *Peaceful Uses of Atomic Energy*, 1956, **11,** 184, United Nations, New York.

DERINGER, M. K., HESTON, W. E., and LORENZ, E. in *Biological Effects of External X and Gamma Radiation*, Part I, (ed. ZIRKLE, R. E.), 1954, N.N.E.S. IV-22B, McGraw-Hill, New York.
DUNN, T. B., *J. Nat. Cancer Institute*, 1954, **14**, 1281.
ESCHENBRENNER, A. B., and MILLER, E. in *Biological Effects of External X and Gamma Radiation*, Part I, (ed. ZIRKLE, R. E.) 1954, N.N.E.S. IV-22B, McGraw-Hill, New York.
EVANS, T. C., *Radiology*, 1948, **50**, 811.
EVANS, T. C., *Nucleonics*, 1949, **4**, 2.
FINKEL, M. P., LISCO, H., and BRUES, A. M., Argonne National Laboratory Report, 1954, ANL 5288.
GORER, P. A., *J. Path. Bact.*, 1940, **50**, 17.
GORER, P. A., *Cancer Research*, 1946, **6**, 470.
HENSHAW, P. S., RILEY, E. F., and STAPLETON G. E., *Radiology*, 1947, **49**, 349.
HENSHAW, P. S., SNIDER, R. S., RILEY, E. F., STAPLETON, G. E., and ZIRKLE, R. E., MDDC 1253, 1946.
LORENZ, E., in *Biological Effects of External X and Gamma Radiation*, Part I (ed. ZIRKLE R. E.), 1954, N.N.E.S. IV-22B, McGraw-Hill, New York.
LORENZ, E., HESTON, W. E., DERINGER, M. K., and ESCHENBRENNER, A. B., *J. Nat. Cancer Institute*, 1946, **6**, 349.
LORENZ, E., HESTON, W. E., ESCHENBRENNER, A. B., and DERINGER, M. K., *Radiology*, 1947, **49**, 274.
LORENZ, E., and JACOBSON L. O., Argonne National Laboratory Report, ANL 4333, 1949.
LORENZ, E., JACOBSON, L. O., HESTON, W. E., SHIMKIN, M., ESCHENBRENNER, A. B., DERINGER, M. K., DONIGER, J., and SCHWEISTHAL, R., in *Biological Effects of External X and Gamma Radiation*, Part I (ed. ZIRKLE, R. E.), 1954, N.N.E.S. IV-22B, McGraw-Hill, New York.
MOLE, R. H., *J. Clin. Path.*, 1954, **7**, 267.
MOLE, R. H., *J. Nat. Cancer Institute*, 1955, **15**, 907.
MOLE, R. H., in International Symposium on Radiobiology, Cambridge, 1955 (ed. MITCHELL, J. S., SMITH, C. L. and HOLMES, B), 1956, Edinburgh.
NEARY, G. J., MUNSON, R. J., and MOLE, R. H., *Nature*, 1953, **171**, 256.
ORR, J. W., *Brit. J. Cancer*, 1947, **1**, 311.
SMITH, F. W., GARDNER, W. U., Li, M. H., and KAPLAN, H., *Cancer Research*, 1949, **9**, 193.
STEWART, H. L. in *Physiopathology of Cancer* (ed. HOMBURGER, F., and FISHMAN, W. H.,) 1953, London.
TANNENBAUM, A., in *Physiopathology of Cancer*, (ed. HOMBURGER, F., and FISHMAN, W. H.), 1953, London.
UPTON, A. C., and FURTH, J., *Proc. Soc. exp. Biol. Med. N.Y.*, 1953, **84**, 255.

CHAPTER IV

RELATIVE BIOLOGICAL EFFICIENCY OF FAST NEUTRONS AND GAMMA RADIATION FOR CHRONIC EXPOSURES

1. RADIATION SOURCES

THE sensitivity of the gonads, both male and female, to fast neutrons has been described in an earlier section. The relatively short irradiation periods, twenty-four hours to five months, required to produce measurable effects at the weekly dose of 6·4 rads made it possible to determine the relative biological efficiency (r.b.e.) of fast neutrons as compared with gamma radiation from ^{60}Co for damage to the gonads of mice. The measurement of the r.b.e. for the killing effects of long-continued irradiation takes much longer since killing effects are so long delayed, and this has necessitated a special experiment the results of which will be reported in due course. For this a similar experimental arrangement was used to that described earlier (Chap. I) but varied so that different fast neutron and gamma dose rates were obtained. Some results of limited exposures in this new arrangement on spleen and testis weight, on female fertility and on blood counts are included in this chapter.

Fast neutron and some gamma ray exposures were obtained as already described. Additional gamma irradiation was provided by multiple sources of ^{60}Co arranged on two horizontal aluminium sheets between which stood the standard aluminium mouse cages like the filling of an English sandwich. Uniformity of dose was good and a variety of dose rates from 80 to 4 r daily were used. These gamma sources were kept in the basement of the laboratory and the environment of the mice was similar to, though not identical with, that of mice being irradiated by fast neutrons.

2. TESTIS WEIGHT

(i) *After a Single Exposure*

The weight of the testis has proved a sensitive indicator of radiation damage by gamma and X rays (Eschenbrenner, Miller and Lorenz, 1948; Kohn and Kallman, 1954) and the decrease in weight four weeks after a single dose of radiation has been used to determine the r.b.e. of X rays and thermal neutrons (Storer and Langham, 1953), and of X rays of different energy (Bane, Tyree, Thompson, Nickson and Shapiro, 1955). The effect of a single dose of 6·5 rads of fast neutrons given in 24 hours has been described earlier (Chap. III, §3 (vi), p. 143). The fresh weight of the testis was also measured at various times after doses of gamma radiation from ^{60}Co and also given in 24 hours. The ratio of the gamma to the fast neutron dose for equal amounts of damage is the r.b.e.

Method

Mice aged 8–10 weeks from a number of litters were earmarked to distinguish the litter of origin and then, just before irradiation, allocated at random to the doses to be used, not more than five to a cage. At the end of the irradiation period the other ear was marked to indicate the dose received and the original litter mates collected together again into one cage where they lived for the few weeks before their testes were weighed. In this way environmental differences between littermates were limited to the twenty-four-hour irradiation period and a maximum of one day before and one day after.

The combined weight of the two testes in each irradiated mouse was expressed as a percentage of the weight in the litter mate control. As Kohn and Kallman (1954) also found, it was necessary to discard some of the observations. Occasionally a mouse had only one testis. Still less frequently one of the testes was much smaller than the other, and it was arbitrarily decided to exclude all mice where the weight of the two testes differed by more than 30 per cent. In addition, for the CBA strain, results were not used when the body weight of a mouse differed by more than 10 per cent from its littermate control at the time the testes were weighed. It was thought preferable to use these objective criteria for discarding results rather than to use Chauvenet's criterion, i.e. to exclude particular observations because they lay outside the range to be expected from the statistics of the group to which they belonged.

The question of whether to express the organ weight as a fraction of the bodyweight will be discussed elsewhere. For C57 Black and F_1 (A×CBA) mice, however, this procedure was preferable since body weight within a litter was more variable than for the CBA strain, and no C57 Black or F_1 mice were excluded because of differences in body weight.

Results

The results for each dose and time-interval after irradiation were combined from several batches of litters irradiated during a period of months. For each of three strains of mice a total of 12 to 16 separate batches of litters were used. In about half of the CBA litters where one mouse received 6·5 rads fast neutrons, one or more mice received one or other of the gamma doses so that a comparison within litters was possible. The other half of these neutron results came from litters where no mouse received gamma radiation, but the results were so similar that the within-litters comparison of gamma radiation and neutrons has not been separately recorded.

The reduction in weight of the testis of CBA mice at various times after gamma irradiation is shown in Fig. 28 together with the results after 6·5 rads of fast neutrons. There was clearly no qualitative

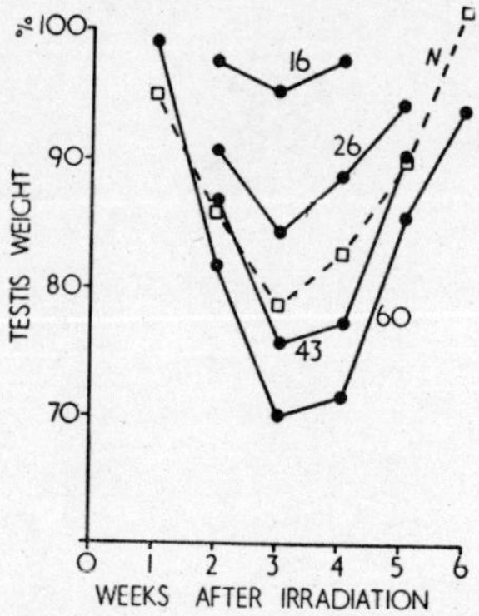

FIG. 28. Testis weight of CBA mice (per cent of litter-mate control) during the six weeks following a single exposure to fast neutrons or gamma radiation.
N = fast neutron dose of *c*. 6·5 rads (cf. Table 55).
Gamma doses shown in figure
Each dose given in 24 hours

difference in the response to the two kinds of radiation. The reduction in weight at three weeks and at four weeks after gamma irradiation was linearly related to the logarithm of the dose (Fig. 29). The mean reduction in testis weight by 6·5 rads of fast neutrons was equal to that expected from 36 r of gamma radiation at three weeks and 33½ r at four weeks. The gamma dose received during the neutron exposure was 1·3 r (Table 55) so that the corrected r.b.e.'s were 5·3 and 5·0 respectively. The weighted average of these was 5·1 (Table 57).

About a year after the gamma exposures additional observations were made three weeks after two other doses of fast neutrons, 2·3 and 13·3 rads, also given in 24 hours.

As long as there was no secular variation in the response of the CBA testis to radiation, (confirmed by unpublished data using X rays), it is permissible to combine the data for all three fast neutron doses. The reduction in testis weight three weeks after fast neutron irradiation when plotted against log (dose) gives a straight line (Fig. 29) with a slope not significantly different from the gamma in Table 57. The r.b.e. is higher, but not significantly higher, than the estimate derived from the single point for 6·5 rads (Table 57).

Data on reduction in testis weight by gamma radiation were also obtained for the other two strains of mice for which neutron effects were also determined. For both C57 Black mice and the F_1 from A×CBA, the time course of reduction in testis weight after irradiation was the same for the two kinds of radiation (Fig. 30). A linear

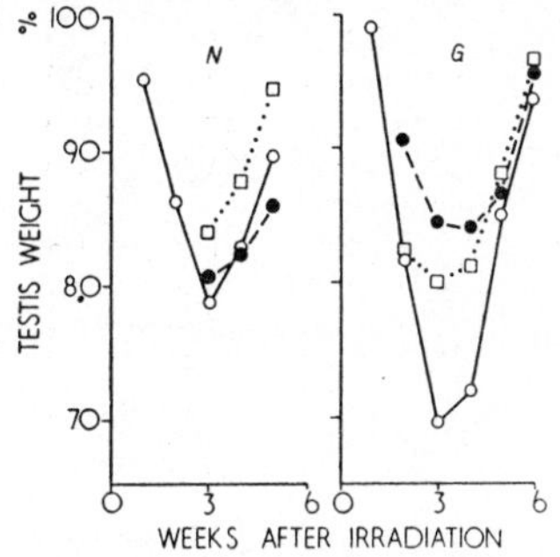

FIG. 30. Testis weight of three genetically different strains of mouse (per cent of litter-mate control) during the six weeks following a single dose of fast neutrons and of gamma radiation.

N = 6·4–6·8 rads of fast neutrons
G = 59–61 r of ^{60}Co
○ CBA
● C57 Black
□ F_1 (A×CBA)

relation between reduction in testis weight and logarithm of dose of gamma radiation was also found at three and four weeks after irradiation. The slopes of the lines for all three mouse strains were statistically indistinguishable. Values of the r.b.e. were calculated from the single point for fast neutron exposure as for CBA mice and are given in Table 57. The difference between the weighted mean values for C57 Black mice and for CBA mice was statistically significant ($P > 0·01$), while the value for the F_1 mice was intermediate and not significantly different from either of the others.

As with CBA mice a dose-response curve for the effect of fast neutrons on C57 Black mice was obtainable if possible secular variation is ignored. Its slope did not differ significantly from that of the gamma line (Fig. 29). The equations for the neutron and gamma lines are given in Table 56 together with the estimate of the relative effectiveness of the two radiations. The r.b.e. obtained in this way is not significantly different from the figures derived from the single contemporaneous fast neutron exposures (Table 57).

TABLE 56

Percentage reduction in testis weight of C57 Black mice after fast neutron and gamma irradiation

	Dose (given in 24 hours) Fast neutron (rads)	Gamma (r)	Time after irradiation — Three weeks: No. of mice	Mean	S.E.	Four weeks: No. of mice	Mean
Gamma exposure	Nil	26	5	1·2	2·2	6	6·7
	Nil	43	5	9·6	0·5	5	9·4
	Nil	59	7	15·4	0·9	7	16·0
	Nil	82	6	21·0	1·0	6	27·7
Fast neutron exposure	2·5	1·2	6	1·7	4·8		
	6·8	1·4	7	19·4	3·4	6†	18·0
	13·3	3·0	4	29·5	1·3		

Equations for response, y, and log(dose), x.			Standard e[rror] of slope
Gamma	Three weeks	$y = -55{\cdot}3+39{\cdot}9x$	4·1
	Four weeks‡	$y = -38{\cdot}9+32{\cdot}6x$	6·7
Fast neutrons	Three weeks	$y = -13{\cdot}8+39{\cdot}1x$	8·0
Combined gamma and fast neutrons	Three weeks	slope = 39·4	4·6

†6·4 rads of fast neutrons, 1·3 r of gamma radiation.

‡ The mean square for deviations from regression was significantly greater than for [...] (P between 0·05 and 0·01).

The difference in the r.b.e. between the different strains for an identical effect was unexpected, but was largely due to the difference in their response to gamma radiation as shown in Fig. 30. It should perhaps be pointed out that the mice were fed and housed identically, irradiated by identical sources and handled identically for determination of testis weight, so that the observed differences in r.b.e. were due solely to genetic differences between the strains.

(ii) *Testis Weight during Chronic Exposure*

Observations were also made on the weight of the testis after various periods of continuous exposure to low levels of gamma and fast neutron radiation (16·5 r and 2·0 rads daily respectively). As before, litter-mates were allocated at random to cages to be placed in each of three tanks and each litter of three was killed on the same day to provide a direct comparison within litters. Since the exposure was a chronic one the mice necessarily lived in the irradiation tanks until the day the testes were examined; litter-mates therefore lived in different cages from each other throughout the experimental period unlike the mice given single doses (p. 157). Four separate batches of mice were used with different starting dates in order to check any possible environmental effect other than irradiation.

The mice used were CBA/H a different subline from that which provided all the other CBA mice used. Partly for this reason and possibly partly because, since these mice were chronically exposed, they were nearly all considerably older than the mice used for the single exposure testis weight experiments, there was a much greater variability of body weight within litters. If the same criteria of exclusion had been used as previously (p. 157) a third of the results would have had to be omitted. The absolute testis weight of controls varied less with age than the testis weight expressed as a proportion of body weight, and was also less variable at any given age. The absolute testis weight without reference to body weight was therefore used as the basis for the experimental comparisons. There was no correlation between body weight and exposure to either fast neutron or gamma radiation at the dose rates used.

The results are given in Table 58. There was a progressive decrease in testis weight in each exposure tank, but the rate of decrease fell

TABLE 58

Testis weight of CBA/H mice (per cent of litter-mate control) during chronic irradiation by low level gamma radiation and fast neutrons

Duration of irradiation (weeks)	No. of litter mate trios	Gamma		Fast neutron	
		Mean	SE	Mean	SE
5	6	82	2	87	3
10	6	82	4	84	2
15	5	73	3	84	6
20	5	69	3	75†	2
25	5	64	3	65	2
30	4	64	2	69	5

† Omitting one result of 26 per cent.

progressively with increase in exposure time. The loss in testis weight was always greater with the gamma exposure of 16·5 r daily than with the fast neutron exposure of 2·0 rads daily. The r.b.e. for chronic exposure was therefore less than 8 and almost certainly not different from the value for a single twenty-four hour exposure (Table 57). Further there was no change in the relative effect of gamma and fast neutron irradiation during the seven months of exposure confirming that the r.b.e. was not altered by extending exposure time.

3. MALE FERTILITY

The method of testing was that described earlier (Chap. III, §3 (iii), p. 132). The gamma irradiations were carried out over about eighteen months and, although the first few months overlapped the last few months of neutron irradiation, the mice irradiated by the two different kinds of radiation were not litter-mates as in some of the comparisons of testis weight. There was nothing to suggest any secular change in radiosensitivity during the course of the experiments on male fertility and some check on this was possible in the mice irradiated by gamma rays.

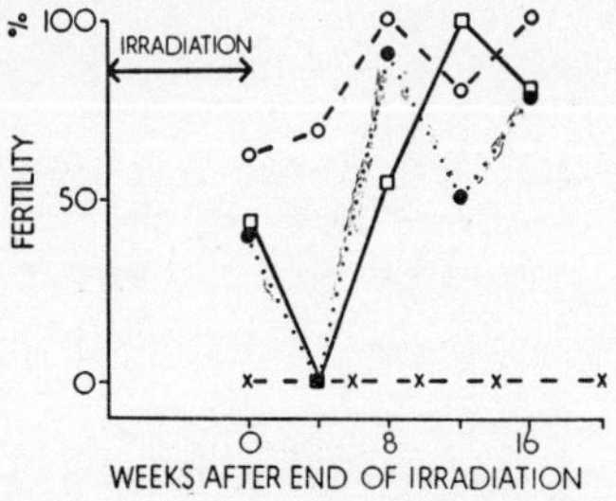

FIG. 31. Fertility of male CBA mice (per cent) after nine weeks' irradiation by fast neutrons or gamma radiation.

□ Fast neutrons 6·4 rads weekly (data from Table 50)
o Gamma radiation 34 r weekly
● Gamma radiation 41 r weekly
× Gamma radiation 84 r weekly

7–10 mice at each point in each gamma group except at time 'O' after 34 r weekly where 14 mice were used.

As in the experiments on testis weight, it was insufficient to confine the comparison of fast neutrons and gamma radiation to measurements of degrees of damage at a single time. The recovery of fertility after removal from irradiation was also followed in order to see if there was any qualitative difference in the effect of the two radiations which might invalidate the determination of the r.b.e. The results on CBA mice are therefore given in two figures comparing the effects of irradiation, for 9 and for 13 weeks respectively, of 6·4 rads weekly of fast neutrons and two or three levels of gamma irradiation, as indicated in the legends.

Fig. 31 shows that 34 r weekly for 9 weeks hardly affected fertility while 84 r weekly not only sterilized the mice by the end of the irradiation period but prevented subsequent recovery. The effect of 6·4 rads weekly of fast neutrons was closely matched by 41 r weekly of gamma radiation: at the end of the nine weeks' irradiation period fertility had fallen to between 40 and 50 per cent, four weeks later fertility was zero but four weeks later still had largely recovered. In each case the size of these first litters after recovery was somewhat smaller than litters produced later in the recovery period. The r.b.e. was thus certainly between 5 and 13 and apparently about 6·5.

Fig. 32 shows that 13 weeks' irradiation at both 32 and 48 r weekly sterilized male CBA mice and that recovery was first evident

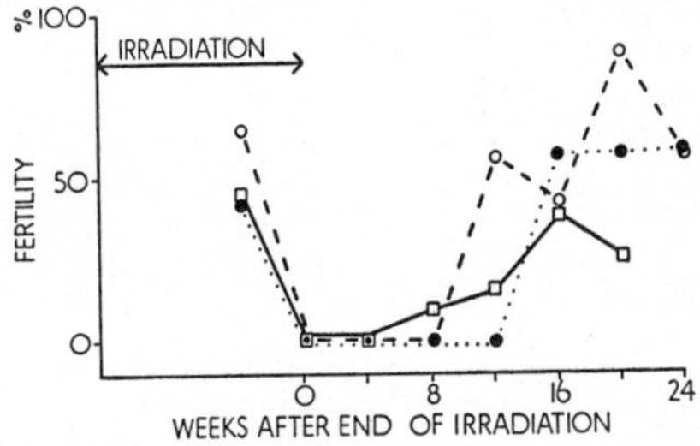

FIG. 32. Fertility of male CBA mice (per cent) after thirteen weeks' irradiation by fast neutrons or gamma radiation.

□ Fast neutrons 6·4 rads weekly (data from Table 50)
○ Gamma radiation 32 r weekly.
● Gamma radiation 48 r weekly.
7–10 mice at each point in each gamma group.

four months after the end of the period of irradiation but was never complete. The effect of 6·4 rads of fast neutrons weekly was similar but an exact r.b.e. cannot be given since there was so little difference between the two levels of gamma irradiation. Further, after doses which allow of only partial recovery it would be expected that uncontrolled environmental differences might have a marked effect in determining the degree of recovery.

Tests of F_1 males from A×CBA showed a considerable increase in radioresistance as compared with CBA males. Complete sterility was produced by nine or thirteen weeks' exposure to 72 r weekly but recovery was complete two months later as judged by the proportion fertile and the size of litter. Since 6·4 rads weekly of fast neutrons did not sterilize after 13 weeks or even 30 weeks (Table 52) the r.b.e. must be less than 11. It is not legitimate however to conclude that the r.b.e. must be less than $(72\times9)/(6{\cdot}4\times30) = 3{\cdot}4$ because this ignores the time factor. This time factor is important: halving the dose rate of gamma irradiation allowed exposure for more than three times as long without producing as much damage. At 39 r weekly there seemed to be a real, if partial reduction in fertility after 25–29 weeks' exposure which would suggest that the r.b.e.

was a little less than 6. The numbers of mice tested during these long exposures were however very small.

4. FEMALE FERTILITY

The method of testing was described earlier (Chap. III, §3 (iii), p. 138). As in the tests of male fertility, most of the female mice given gamma irradiation were irradiated after the conclusion of the neutron irradiations, but again there was nothing to suggest any secular change in radiosensitivity and a little evidence against any such change.

Damage to the ovaries of mice is not followed by recovery (Deringer, Heston and Lorenz, 1954), so that the only possible comparison between gamma and neutron radiation was in the degree of damage produced. It was found by Deringer *et al.* (1954) that the degree of ovarian damage by daily gamma irradiation was the same whether the daily dose was given in 1, 8 or 24 hours. Similarly after fast neutron irradiation the effect was the same whether the weekly dose was given continuously or on only one day in seven (Table 53). Nevertheless, we found that the total dose required to produce a given degree of damage altered with the overall exposure time.

As already described, the radiation damage was measured by the proportion of mice made completely infertile or by the size of the first litter. The total number of young produced, or reproductive capacity, is not easily used as a measure of effect since the expected figure for normal controls clearly varies with the age of the animal

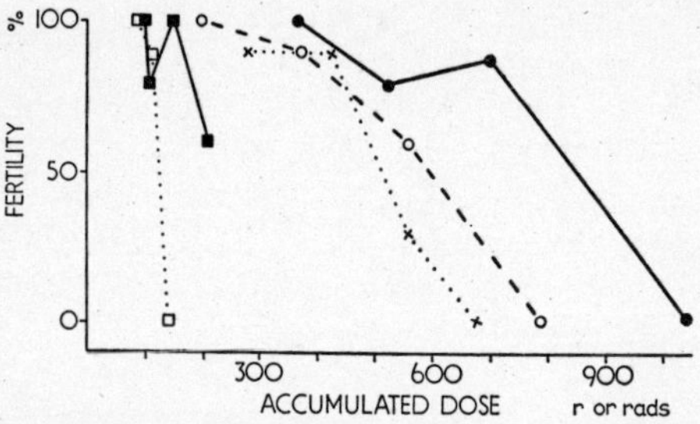

FIG. 33. Fertility of female CBA mice (per cent) and accumulated dose of radiation (r or rads): chronic irradiation by fast neutrons and by gamma radiation.

	No. of mice at a point
■ Fast neutrons 15 rads weekly	10
□ Fast neutrons 6·4 rads weekly	8–9
● Gamma radiation 74 r weekly	8–12
○ Gamma radiation 43 r weekly	10
× Gamma radiation 33 r weekly	10

when first mated, and animals irradiated at different levels of daily dose are likely to differ widely in this respect.

Data for CBA mice are given in Figs. 33 and 35 and show, for both

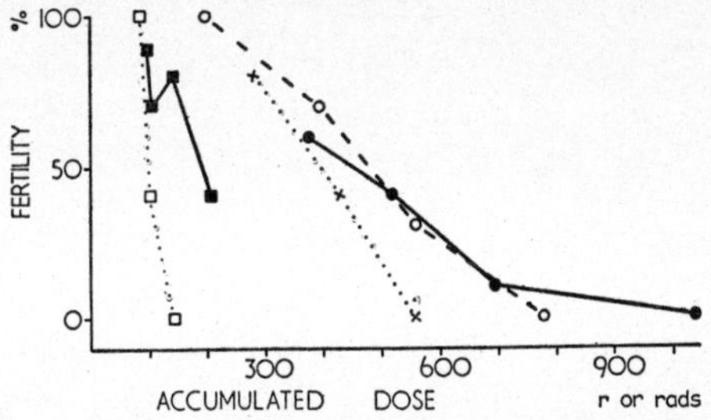

FIG. 34. Accumulated dose of radiation (r or rads) and fertility of female CBA mice (per cent) ignoring litters conceived in the first 20 days after the end of the irradiation.
Symbols as in Fig. 33.

gamma and fast neutron irradiation, and for both criteria of damage, that the amount of radiation required to produce a given degree of damage was reduced as the weekly dose was reduced, i.e. as the

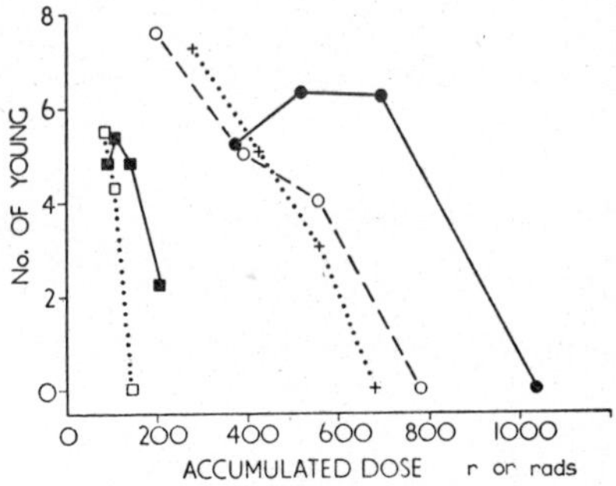

FIG. 35. Size of first litter in female CBA mice and accumulated dose of radiation (r or rads); chronic irradiation by fast neutrons and by gamma radiation. Mice and symbols as in Fig. 33.

exposure time was increased. There are at least two possible reasons for this. One is that with increasing age the ovary may become more radiosensitive; the duration of irradiation at the lower dose-rates brought the mice near to the age when natural fertility begins to be impaired anyway. Secondly it is usually thought that an ovary so damaged that no more new follicles will be formed may still produce fertilizable ova for a short time. The shorter the irradiation period (i.e. the higher the dose rate) the more likely is it that such ova will be detected by the method used here of mating immediately on removal from the irradiation field. This second factor may perhaps be obviated by ignoring all litters conceived within the first twenty

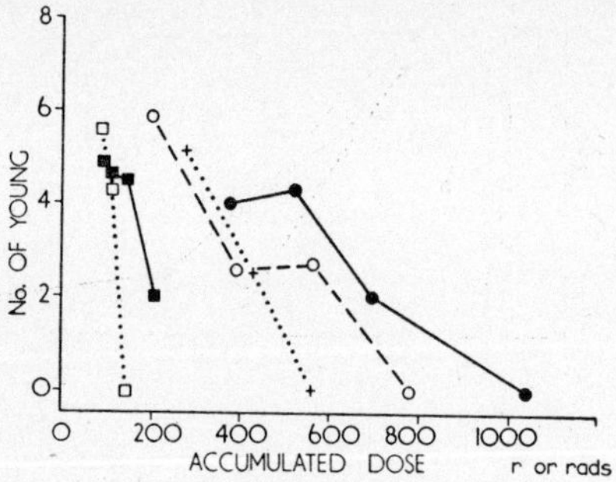

FIG. 36. Accumulated dose of radiations (r or rads) and size of first litter in female CBA mice ignoring litters conceived in the first 20 days after the end of the irradiation.

Mice and symbols as in Fig. 34.

days. The dose-response curve for ovarian damage is then shifted along the dose axis but the effect of exposure time is still visible (Figs. 34 and 36).

The importance of exposure time to the determination of the r.b.e. is that a comparison of two radiations can properly be made only

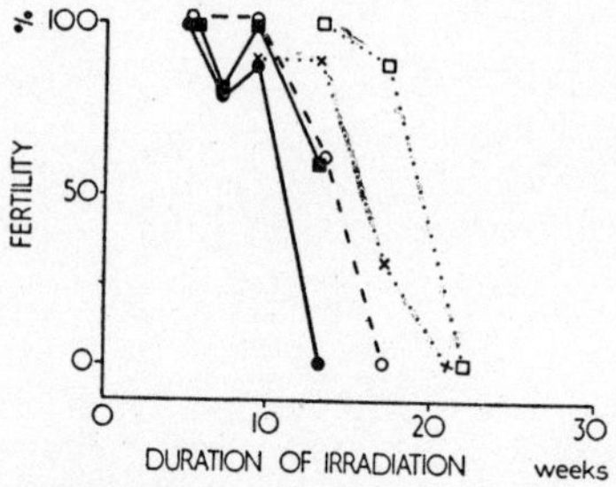

FIG. 37. Fertility of female CBA mice (per cent) and duration of irradiation (weeks): chronic irradiation by fast neutrons and by gamma radiation.

Mice and symbols as in Fig. 33.

The effect of 6·4 rads weekly □ was less than that of 33 r weekly × making the r.b.e. less than 5. The effect of 15 rads weekly ■ was closely similar to that of 43 r weekly ○ giving an r.b.e. of 3.

if the time taken to produce the same degree of biological damage is about the same. In Figs. 37 and 38 the degree of biological damage in CBA mice is plotted against time of exposure for two fast neutron dose rates and three gamma dose rates. The results give clear limits to the possible values of the r.b.e., as indicated in the legends to the figures, and the best value is probably about 3.

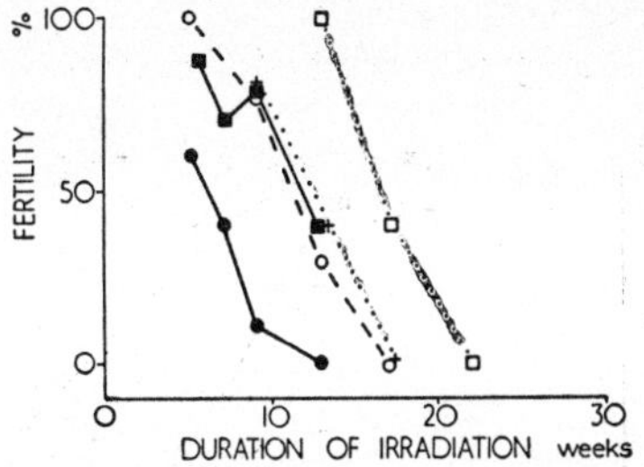

FIG. 38. Duration of irradiation (weeks) and fertility of female CBA mice ignoring litters conceived in the first 20 days after the end of the irradiation. Mice and symbols as in Fig. 34.

The effect of 15 rads weekly ■ was closely similar to that of 33 and of 43 r weekly × and o giving an r.b.e. of about 2½.

The dose required to reduce fertility by a half (under the conditions of this experiment) may be estimated visually from the data in Fig. 33. In Fig. 39 this is plotted against log (dose rate) for both fast neutrons and gamma radiation. It is clear that parallel straight lines

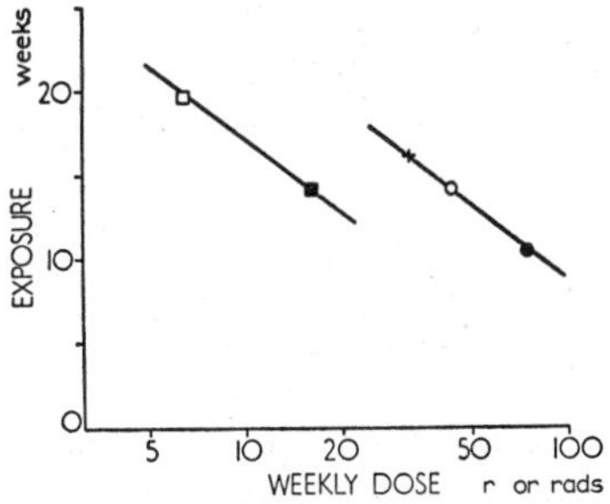

FIG. 39. Duration of exposure (weeks) needed to halve the fertility of female CBA mice and weekly dose (logarithmic scale) of fast neutrons and of gamma radiation.

The neutron line is on the left, the gamma line on the right. Mice and symbols as in Fig. 33.

may be drawn through the two sets of points and that the intercept between the lines gives an r.b.e. of 2·7.

Data for the two other strains of mouse were also obtained. F_1 (A×CBA) females needed over 700 r of gamma radiation at 70 r weekly to halve their fertility, much more than the 150 r at half the dose rate needed for C57 Black Mice. CBA mice were intermediate in sensitivity. Data for F_1 mice at two neutron levels and three gamma levels of irradiation are given in Fig. 40. Exposure time is again seen to be important. When the daily dose of gamma radiation was reduced four and a half times, the dose required to sterilize was reduced by a third, and the same sort of change was

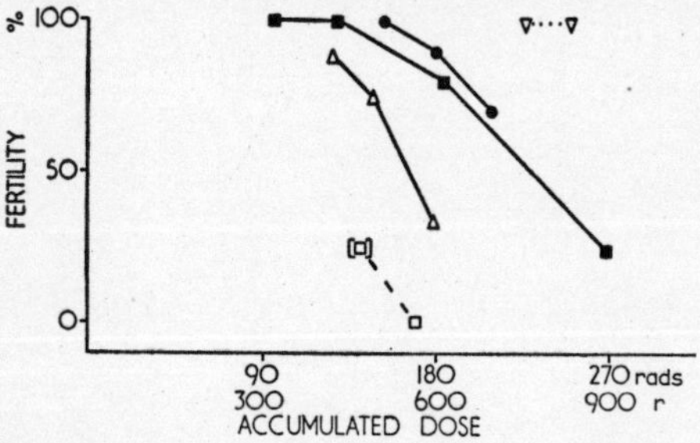

FIG. 40. Dose of radiation (r or rads) and fertility of female F_1 (A×CBA) mice after chronic irradiation by fast neutrons and by gamma radiation. Fast neutron and gamma doses are shown on a scale of 1 : 3·3.

		No. of mice to a point
■	Fast neutrons 15 rads weekly	5–10
□	Fast neutrons 6·4 rads weekly	4–8
▽	Gamma radiation 110 r weekly	7–10
●	Gamma radiation 70 r weekly	10
△	Gamma radiation 16 r weekly	8–9

The data from 15 rads weekly would have been superimposed on those from 70 r weekly if the dose scales had been in the ratio 1 : 3·6.

clearly true of fast neutron exposure too. The effect of a weekly dose of as little as 16 r of gamma radiation was definite. The r.b.e. is about 4 if the effect of exposure time is ignored, or about 3 when allowance is made for exposure time.

CBA and F_1 female mice, when mated, conceived in the next ten days or so, as a rule, if they were ever going to be fertile and this was true whether they were normal or irradiated. On the other hand, C57 Black mice commonly took up to 2 months to produce their first litter, sometimes more than 3 months. Normal mice showed the same kind of behaviour though not so extremely as irradiated mice. The males used for testing C57 Black females were rotated every fortnight amongst the cages under test so that immaturity or infertility of the C57 male was not the cause. However, litters conceived late were normal in size in control mothers but much smaller in irradiated mothers, and the mean size of the first litter produced has been the most useful criterion of radiation damage in C57 Black mice. Data for two gamma dose rates and two neutron dose rates are given in Fig. 41 and suggest that r.b.e. is also about 3. The effect of 16 r weekly is rather more obvious in C57 Black mice than in the F_1.

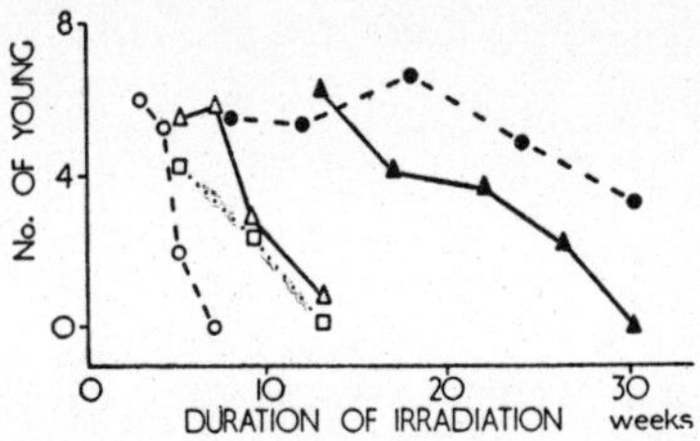

FIG. 41. Duration of irradiation (weeks) and size of first litter in female C57 Black mice after chronic irradiation by fast neutrons and by gamma radiation.

	No. of mice to a point
□ Fast neutrons 6·4 rads weekly	4–8
▲ Fast neutrons 2·4 rads weekly	4–5
○ Gamma radiation 31 r weekly	10–15
△ Gamma radiation 16 r weekly	9–10
● Unirradiated controls examined at different ages to correspond with various durations of irradiation. These litter-mate controls were virgin mice mated for the first time at the times indicated, just as were the irradiated mice.	

The r.b.e.'s for effects of gamma and fast neutron irradiation on female fertility have been derived from the dose measurements 'in air' without making any allowance for the attenuation of the radiations within the body of the mouse. For the gamma radiation this can be disregarded. For fast neutrons of the energy employed it has been shown that the mean dose in the mouse is likely to have been about 75 per cent of the 'in air' dose (Chap. I, §12, p. 27). The situation of the ovaries within the mouse is such that the fast neutron dose they receive should approximate to this mean dose. The quoted r.b.e.'s for effects on female fertility may therefore be too low by one third, i.e. they should perhaps be as high as 4 for the three mouse strains examined. On the other hand with an r.b.e. of this magnitude the additional dose due to the gamma contamination of the fast neutrons (Tables 1 and 19) becomes significant, and if this is taken into account the r.b.e.'s should be reduced by about 10 per cent. Since these two sources of systematic error partially neutralized each other it was considered preferable to ignore them both when calculating the r.b.e.'s for damage to female fertility.

(ii) *The Effect of Age on the Radiation Sensitivity of Female Fertility*

As shown by Figs. 33 and 40 the total dose required to damage female fertility decreased as exposure time was prolonged. This could have been due either to a real increase in the damaging action of radiation as the dose rate was reduced or to an increase in radio-sensitivity with increasing age. A supplementary experiment was carried out to decide this question.

F_1 (A×CBA) females were used in preference to other strains because they do not become naturally infertile till after they are a year old and more time was thus available in which to do the experiment. Batches of litters were distributed between cages as usual and placed in a gamma exposure tank at the age of three, six or nine months. The cages were left in the tank for varying periods from four to eight weeks, depending on age, and removed and tested for fertility as usual by continuous mating with removal of litters as born. The F_1 females carried the milk factor and because they developed mammary tumours, some of the older mice had inevitably to be discarded either before or during irradiation or too soon after mating for results to be usable.

The results are given in Table 59. They show clearly that the older the animal the smaller the dose of radiation required to reduce fertility and reproductive capacity. Even if allowance is made for the natural reduction in reproductive capacity with ageing, it still

TABLE 59

Mean number of young produced by F_1 (A×CBA) mice of different ages in the first 100 days immediately following the end of exposure to gamma radiation (mean weekly dose 105r)

Duration of irradiation (weeks)	Age at onset of irradiation (weeks) 10–12	26–28	40–42
4		16·3 (3)	10·3 (4)
5	24·5 (8)	12·8 (5)	8·2 (6)
6			0·9 (7)†
7	15·5 (10)	8·7 (7)	
8	12·3 (8)		

Controls: Age at start of test of fertility (weeks) 38	48	52	56
16·0 (7)	10·4 (7)	9·0 (8)	7·7 (7)

Number of mice tested in parentheses.

† Only 4 out of 7 fertile. All other groups 100 per cent fertile except controls aged 52 weeks where one mouse was infertile.

appears as if the older the animal the less the amount of radiation needed to produce a given amount of damage, e.g. to halve the reproductive capacity as compared with controls of the same age.

5. HAEMATOLOGICAL CHANGES

As described earlier, a weekly dose rate of 6·4 rads of fast neutrons scarcely affected the white count during nine months' exposure (Table 44). A weekly dose rate of 16 rads reduced the white count to less than half that of litter-mate controls examined at the same time (cf. Chap. III, §3 (i), p. 129). Other litter-mates exposed to 110 r weekly of gamma radiation showed a closely similar reduction in total white cell count (Fig. 42). The r.b.e. for this effect would thus be about 7.

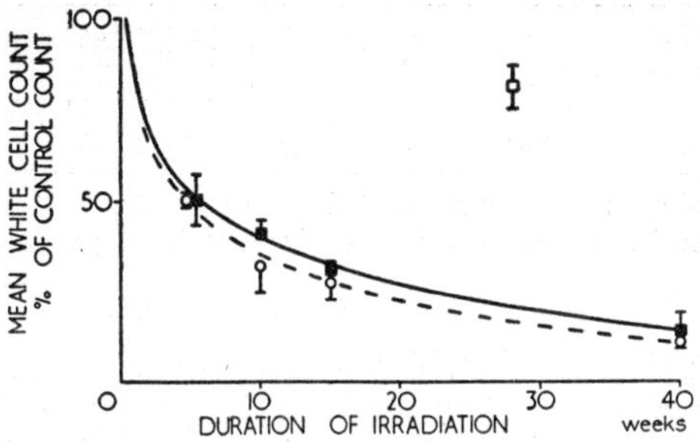

FIG. 42. Duration of irradiation (weeks) and total white blood cell count of irradiated CBA mice (per cent of litter-mate control).

■ Fast neutrons 16 rads weekly
□ Fast neutrons 6·4 rads weekly
○ Gamma radiation 110 r weekly

The curves are theoretical ones assuming the percentage blood count to be proportional to log (duration of irradiation in weeks).

The relative effect of the fast neutron and gamma exposures was the same throughout the 40 week exposure period suggesting that the r.b.e. did not change as the duration of irradiation increased. The heterophils and lymphocytes were depressed to about the same degree by both kinds of radiation so that the r.b.e. for leukopenia and lymphopenia were the same and also about 7.

6. WEIGHT OF SPLEEN AND THYMUS

The weight of the thymus and the spleen, like that of the testis, has been used for estimations of the r.b.e. of different radiations (Harris and Brennan, 1952; Worman, Turney and Lotz, 1954; Jordan, Clark and Vogel, 1956). Unlike the testis, however, the other two organs are relatively insensitive and were not affected by 6·4 rads of fast neutrons weekly (Table 45). At the higher weekly dose of 16 rads there was a small reduction in weight of both thymus and spleen and in Table 60 this is compared with the effect of 110 r

TABLE 60

Mean weight ± S.E. of spleen and thymus (per cent of litter-mate controls) during chronic irradiation by fast neutrons (N) and by gamma radiation (G)

Duration of irradiation (weeks)	Fast neutron exposure: Fast neutrons (rads)	Fast neutron exposure: Gamma contamination (r)	Gamma dose (r)	Spleen N	Spleen G	Thymus N	
5	77 (5)	30	560 (6)	81±4	71±4	89±6	87
10	158 (8)	57	1120 (8)	70±3	68±6	91±12	77
15	237 (5)	83	1600 (5)	73±3	70±3	84±8	92
40	630 (4)	230	4400 (2)	59±8	59±11		

The fresh weight of each organ was divided by the body weight before dividing b corresponding ratio for the control. The numbers in parentheses give the number of litter pairs used.

weekly of gamma radiation. The effects of the two kinds of radiation were indistinguishable after the first five weeks, giving an r.b.e. of about 7. It is interesting that the spleen was affected proportionately more than the thymus by both kinds of chronic irradiation, the opposite of what was found for single doses of X rays by Kallman and Kohn (1955), but the same as was found after daily X irradiation of rats by Brues, Sacher and France (1947).

7. DISCUSSION

When the biologically damaging effects of fast neutrons and other kinds of radiation were first compared, the interest of the results lay mainly in the light they might throw on the relation between physical and biological events on the submicroscopic scale (Lea, 1946). It was implicitly assumed, perhaps, that the relative biological efficiency observed for some kind of effect, for example, chromosome breakage, would be roughly the same wherever it was observed, and that the more complex effects might be interpreted in terms of these 'simpler' observations. Boag (1953) made a valuable and critical review of all the information then available and considered the defects, physical and biological, which complicated the interpretation of many of the reported experiments. So far, the radiobiological data (his Class 2) have not proved helpful in assessing the damaging effects on mammals, which have had to be directly investigated by radio-toxicological experiments (Boag's Class 1).

From the radio-toxicological viewpoint the most important question was whether the r.b.e. varied with the dose rate at which the radiation was administered. Evans (1948 and 1949) had suggested that the r.b.e. of fast neutrons to X radiation for damage to mammals might increase as the daily dose decreased to maximum permissible levels and indeed that this might be expected from what was known of the radiobiology of these two kinds of radiation.

Our own observations have not confirmed this suggestion of Evans. None of the values of the r.b.e. for chronic exposures were high. The r.b.e. for impairment of female fertility in CBA mice was unchanged at the low figure of 3 when the duration of irradiation was increased from 10 to 20 weeks. The r.b.e. for reduction in testis weight by a twenty-four hours' exposure was not significantly different from the r.b.e. for up to seven months' exposure at a much smaller dose rate or from the r.b.e. for impairment in male fertility by a nine weeks' exposure.

The importance of dose rate has been emphasized by Boag (1953). Apart from the way in which dose rate affects interaction of the immediate products of the primary physical events, and hence their biological effect, exposure time may be a quantitatively important factor because biological systems with the capacity for recovery can only recover at limited rates, which may be sufficient to balance damage at low dose rates but insufficient at high dose rates. To these may be added a third factor, the interaction of radiation and of ageing of the biological system, which is especially relevant when radiotoxicological experiments are carried out at the lowest possible dose rate in order to get as near as may be to maximum permissible levels. The existence of this interaction was demonstrated by Carter, Lyon and Phillips (1954) when examining the effect of gamma irradiation on the fertility of male CBA mice, and also by us when examining female fertility (Chap. IV, §4 (ii) p. 172).

When discussing experiments with chronic irradiation these last two factors must always be borne in mind because they can work together to produce apparently contradictory results. Thus, as the exposure time is prolonged, the dose required to produce an effect may initially increase and then decrease. Reducing the dose rate and prolonging exposure time decreased damage to male fertility (Deringer, Heston and Lorenz, 1954 and our experiments on F_1 mice (Chap. IV, §3, p. 165)). In both these experiments hybrid mice were used and the testes of such mice have a greater rate of recovery after single doses of radiation than some, if not all, pure strains (unpublished observations of the authors). When mice were used with a lower rate of recovery from radiation damage and an earlier onset of natural infertility, such as CBA mice, not only was complete sterilization produced by a smaller total dose, but prolonging the exposure time led not to an increase but to a further reduction in the damaging dose (Carter *et al.*, 1954). This was due to the effects of ageing; in the experiments of Carter *et al.* (1954) fertility was assessed after 25 weeks of irradiation at 8·0 r weekly at an age when the natural fertility of the unirradiated controls was beginning to diminish.

The characteristic response of testis weight to chronic irradiation was found by Eschenbrenner, Miller and Lorenz (1948), and in pattern is very similar to the response of the white blood cells (Fig. 42). Clearly the testis behaves as envisaged above: if the daily dose is not too high the weight of the testis is maintained nearly constant in the face of continued irradiation because of an approximate balance between continued damage and continued repair. To determine the relative biological efficiency of two kinds of radiation it would be simplest to make the comparison after the steady state had been reached. The only previously published experimental data appear to be those of Evans (1948) where the testis was weighed after weekly doses of 7 N of fast neutrons and of 55 r and 75 r X rays. The reported testis weight/body weight ratios were the average for mice variously exposed for periods of 1 to 15 weeks (Evans, 1955, personal communication), and thus do not give the steady state levels (cf. Table 58). After the 15 weeks irradiation period the testis weight/body weight ratio was of the order of 20 per cent of the controls for all radiation groups (Evans, 1955, personal communication). With such gross damage the comparison of neutron and X rays is not sensitive but whether these figures or Evans's published ones are used the r.b.e. (r/rad) is about 5 (one N = 2 rad) agreeing well with our own value for a single exposure of twenty four hours' duration.

Male fertility was also examined by Evans (1948) at the same dose rates. Ignoring any effect of exposure time and comparing the accumulated doses needed to produce complete sterility gave an r.b.e. of 17 assuming 1 N = 2 rads (Evans, 1949). However, complete sterility was reached after 5–8 weeks' irradiation by fast neutrons and after 12–31 weeks of X radiation. For hybrid mice such a difference in exposure time would exaggerate the difference in accumulated dose (see earlier in this discussion) and it is clear that Evans's figure for this r.b.e. must be an over-estimate. Since the time needed to produce complete sterility was longer at weekly doses of 75 r of

X rays than of 7 N or 14 rads of neutrons, the r.b.e. (r/rad) must have been more than 5. From the data available it is not possible to say whether the figure was significantly different from that for reduction in testis weight or what its likely limits may have been.

Recovery factors are believed not to complicate experiments on female fertility. The data of Evans (1948) on the oestrus cycle showed that 7 N or 14 rads weekly of neutrons produced complete anoestrus earlier than 55 r weekly of X rays so that the r.b.e. (r/rad) was greater than 4. The comparison of total dose to produce the same effect gave an r.b.e. (r/rad) of 7, but our experiments have shown that it is misleading to make such a comparison of doses accumulated at weekly doses differing by nearly twofold in the time needed to produce the same degree of damage. If, because of increasing exposure time (radiation-age interaction), the total dose needed to produce an effect was reduced, then the r.b.e. as determined by comparison of total doses would be still further increased. The end point used in our experiments on female fertility was different from Evans's and our estimations of the r.b.e. are definitely less than his.

Thus where comparisons can be made (tests of male and female fertility) the values for the r.b.e. obtained by Evans (1948) seem to have been higher than those obtained by us, even when allowance is made for complicating biological factors and for differences in effectiveness of the X rays and gamma radiation used as baselines. The differences may lie merely in the use of different mouse stocks; genetic differences have been shown to affect the r.b.e. for testis damage (Chap. IV, §2, p. 162). However, there may also have been some relevant difference in dose measurement, energy of neutrons, or proportion of the day free from radiation. Differences in distribution of the fast neutron dose through the body of the mouse do not seem to be responsible for the difference between our estimates and those of Evans. His cyclotron neutrons were more energetic than the fission neutrons used by us, and even with these less energetic neutrons the dose to the ovary was little less than the quoted 'in air' dose (Chap. IV, §4, p. 171).

The manner in which the white blood-cell count responds to chronic irradiation by fast neutrons (Fig. 42) is another good illustration of the importance of recovery rate. There was little change after more than six months at 6·4 rads weekly, but at a dose rate two and a half times greater a substantial reduction after five weeks' irradiation and a progressively slower decrease during the subsequent 35 weeks. To ignore dose rate and calculate accumulated doses which did or did not produce a change in white count could lead to erroneous conclusions. It is clear that at 6·4 rads weekly the body could compensate for the radiation damage almost as fast as it was produced whereas at 16 rads weekly the balance between rate of repair and rate of damage was struck at a subnormal level. The weight of the spleen and the thymus depended on dose rate in a similar way (Tables 45 and 60).

It was, however, primarily a comparison of acute killing effects after single doses with shortening of life after chronic exposures which suggested that protraction increased the r.b.e. Evans (1948) found the same r.b.e. for single large doses and for repeated doses large enough to kill in three weeks, but for chronic exposure killing in six months a larger r.b.e., perhaps twice as large. Henshaw, Riley and Stapleton (1947) found the r.b.e. to increase four times when single large doses were compared with daily doses killing in six months or so.

It is probably relevant that in experiments with continuous irradiation till death, the amount of radiation required to kill is always exaggerated and that the unnecessary or wasted radiation is proportionately largest with dose rates which kill at between six months and a year after the start (Mole, 1955). This biological factor may not be quantitatively the same for neutrons and gamma radiation and differences in the wasted proportion of continued radiation might put a different interpretation on the facts recorded by Henshaw *et al.* (1947) and Evans (1948).

Further, their methods of determining the r.b.e. may be open to criticism. As Evans (1948) showed, a change in the method of analysing the data could alter the r.b.e. nearly threefold. His method, of comparing the accumulated doses at the 50 per cent survival point, assumes that this dose is independent of exposure time, which is certainly untrue. Henshaw *et al.* (1947) drew the curve relating percentage reduction in median life span to dose rate of fast neutrons and interpolated the reduction in life span by 8·6 r daily of gamma radiation to find its equivalent in neutrons. The shape of the curve was such that its slope was steeper, and hence the errors of interpolation greater, the lower the daily dose. The value of the r.b.e. depended almost entirely on the particular figures of 24 and 16 per cent for the shortening of life by 8·6 r daily and by 0·115 n or 0·2 rads daily. Apart from the fact that the r.b.e. depended essentially on only two experimental points, the criterion of effect was the time taken for half the animals in a group to die as determined by inspection of the survival curve. The life-spans of all but the median animal were thus ignored in assessing the results.

Through the courtesy of Dr. A. Hollaender and Dr. G. E. Stapleton the individual survival times for each animal were obtained and the data analysed by the method described above (Chap. III, §2 (i),

p. 100) of calculating the excess mortality of irradiated groups over the control group. The excess mortalities thus derived are shown in Fig. 43 and strongly suggest a systematic change in excess mor-

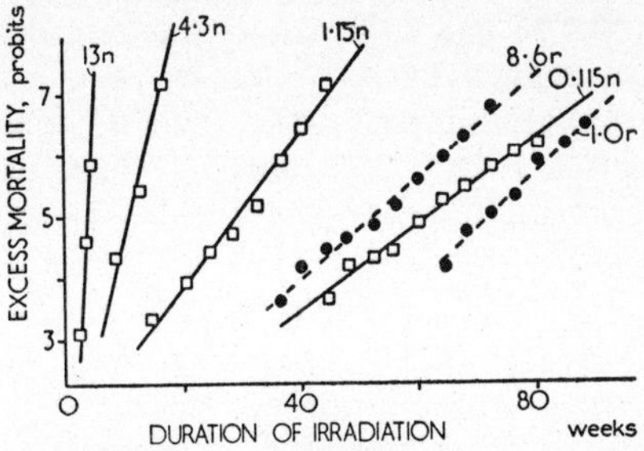

FIG. 43. Duration of irradiation (weeks) and excess mortality over controls (probits) for chronic irradiation by fast neutrons and by gamma radiation (data of Henshaw *et al.*, 1946, 1947).

□ Fast neutrons ● Gamma radiation

Daily dose shown by each line, in 'n' units for fast neutrons, in r for gamma radiation.

tality with dose rate. When the duration of irradiation corresponding to an excess mortality of 50 per cent was plotted against dose rate on a logarithmic scale a reasonable straight line was obtained

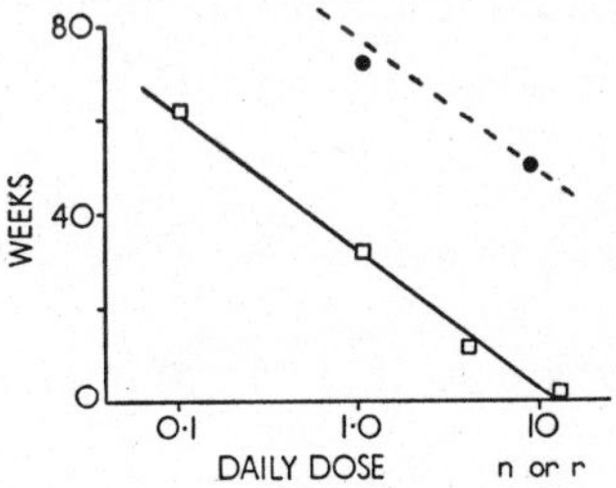

FIG. 44. Daily dose (log scale) and duration of irradiation corresponding to 50 per cent excess mortality for chronic irradiation by fast neutrons and by gamma radiation.

Data from Fig. 43. Symbols as in Fig. 43.

The line through the 8·6 r daily gamma point is drawn parallel to the line through the neutron points. The horizontal intercept between the lines is 1·6 giving an r.b.e. (r/n) of 40, or r.b.e. (r/rad) of 20, if 1 n = 2 rad.

for each kind of radiation (Fig. 44), and it became possible to make use of all the neutron and gamma dose levels in determining the r.b.e. The excess mortality produced by 1 r daily of gamma radiation was small and uncertain. If this group is disregarded the r.b.e.

(r/n) was 20, (i.e. r.b.e. r/rad was 10), about half that determined by the method of Henshaw *et al.* (1947). And, if the data from the 1 r group are included, there is nothing to indicate that the r.b.e. increases with decreasing dose rate for, if this were so, the gamma and neutron lines in Fig. 44 should have diverged more and more as the dose rates decreased.

It might be thought that the discrepancies would be resolved if the r.b.e. for single and for multiple exposures were different and if the r.b.e. for multiple exposures did not vary with exposure time. The results of Evans (1948) do not support this suggestion for he found the same r.b.e. for single acute exposures and for daily exposures killing in three weeks and a larger r.b.e. for daily exposures killing in six months. The question of whether the r.b.e. systematically increases with decreasing dose rate is only likely to be answered by an experiment using several dose rates of each of the two kinds of radiation so that some comparison may be made of the sort attempted in Figs. 39 and 44. To compare the r.b.e. for single killing doses and for some one dose rate of chronic irradiation may be misleading as Evans (1948) pointed out.

In spite of the wide variety of experimental arrangements and mouse stocks used in work on duration-of-life irradiation, there is a remarkable general similarity about the results obtained by all investigators when per cent shortening of life span as compared

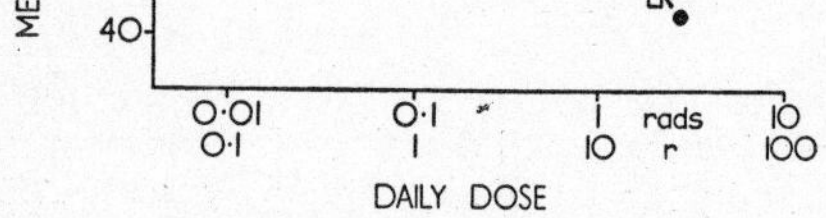

FIG. 45. Daily dose (log scale) and mean survival time (per cent of control) after chronic irradiation by fast neutrons and by gamma radiation (experiments of several authors).

■——■ Fast neutrons: this paper
●---● Fast neutrons: Evans (1948, 1949)
□——□ Fast neutrons: Henshaw *et al.* (1946, 1947)
×——× Gamma radiation: Henshaw *et al.* (1946, 1947)
o······o Gamma radiation: Lorenz *et al.* (1947, 1954)

The fast neutron and gamma scales are in the ratio of 1 to 10, so that if the r.b.e. were, 10 the data should coincide.

with the controls is used as the measure of effect. This is true even though the life spans of the control groups varied by 100 per cent. In Fig. 45 are plotted the results of three experiments with fast neutrons and two with gamma radiation by four separate groups of investigators. It would appear as if an r.b.e. of 10 for chronic killing effects in mice must be near the truth. It should be remembered however that the dose rate is plotted logarithmically and that the scale of the figure is such that the spread of the data corresponds to a twofold uncertainty either way in this ratio.

In confirmation of the greater sensitivity of the gonads than any other organ in mice, it may be seen from Fig. 45 that daily doses of 2–3 r daily of gamma radiation appeared to shorten life by about 10 per cent, a shortening which was just significant in the experiment of Lorenz *et al.* (Sampford 1952). The same daily dose of gamma radiation was shown to reduce female fertility to a half by the end of the first or second third of the reproductive span (C57 Black and F_1 mice respectively, Figs. 41 and 40) and to cause loss of half the sperm-producing elements of the testis in four to five months (Table 58).

The production of cataracts is undoubtedly a form of radiation damage where neutrons have a high r.b.e. compared with X or gamma radiation (Ham, 1954) but there is little information about effects of chronic irradiation. Even with cataract, dose rate has an effect so that, as with the testis, the proper comparison is between dose rates producing equal amounts of damage, not between total accumulated doses. At 6·4 rads weekly of fast neutrons grossly obvious cataracts did not appear for over a year and it is arguable how far they were due directly to the effects of radiation on the lens.

A very brief abstract of some of this work has already been published (Mole, Munson and Neary, 1955). The values quoted for the relative biological efficiencies have since been altered following the revision of the fast neutron dose rate calculations (Chap. II, §7 (i), p. 41).

8. SUMMARY

(1) When a tissue is able to recover from radiation damage it may be wrong to calculate the r.b.e. for chronic irradiation from the total accumulated doses required to produce an effect. The proper comparison is between the dose rates which produce an effect of the same degree at the same time after the start of irradiation.

(2) As female mice aged, their fertility became more easily damaged by irradiation. Thus when experiments are carried out at

low daily doses the dose-response relation may depend on exposure time because of an interaction of ageing and radiation. Misleading comparisons are possible if this is ignored.

(3) No qualitative difference was found between gamma radiation and fast neutrons in their effects on the weight of the testis, spleen and thymus, male fertility, female fertility and the white blood cell count.

(4) The r.b.e. of fast neutrons compared with ^{60}Co gamma radiation for reduction in testis weight after a 24 hour exposure was 5·1, 6·2 and 9·7 for three genetically different strains of mouse. The extreme values were significantly different from each other.

(5) The r.b.e. as measured by reduction in testis weight appeared to be about the same whether single twenty-four hour exposures were given or continuous daily irradiation for up to seven months.

(6) The r.b.e. for impairment of male fertility by chronic irradiation was about 6 or 7 in CBA mice.

(7) The r.b.e. for impairment of female fertility by chronic irradiation was about 3 in each of three genetically different strains of mouse, which varied severalfold in their absolute sensitivity to radiation.

(8) The r.b.e. for reduction in spleen weight and in the white cell count of the peripheral blood was about 7.

(9) Comparisons of fast neutron and gamma irradiation were made for exposure times from 24 hours to 9 months. Within this range there was no evidence that alterations in exposure time or dose rate altered the r.b.e., and published evidence to the contrary is critically examined and found wanting.

(10) A comparison of all available information on mortality of chronically irradiated mice suggests that the r.b.e. for this effect is likely to be about 10.

(11) Evidence was obtained that the gonads are the most sensitive organs in the mouse to chronic irradiation at very low dose rates.

REFERENCES

Bane, H. N., Tyree, E. B., Thompson, P. A., Nickson, J. J., and Shapiro, G., *Radiation Research*, 1955, **3**, 213.

Boag, T. W., The relative biological efficiency of different ionizing radiations, 1953, National Bureau of Standards Report, 2946, Washington.

Brues, A. M., Sacher, G. A., and France, H. O., Argonne National Laboratory Report CH-3825, 1947.

Carter, T. C., Lyon, M. F., and Phillips, R. J. S., *Brit. J. Radiology*, 1954, **27**, 418.

DERINGER, M. K., HESTON, W. E., and LORENZ, E. in *Biological Effects of External X and Gamma Radiation*, Part I, (ed. ZIRKLE, R. E.), 1954, N.N.E.S. IV-22B, McGraw-Hill, New York.

ESCHENBRENNER, A. B., MILLER, E., and LORENZ, E., *J. Nat. Cancer Institute*, 1948, **9**, 133.

EVANS, T. C., *Radiology*, 1948, **50**, 811.

EVANS, T. C., *Nucleonics*, 1949, **4**, 2.

HAM, W. T., *Arch. Ophthalmol.*, 1953, **39**, 285.

HARRIS, P. S., and BRENNAN, J. T., Los Alamos Scientific Laboratory Report, 1952, LA-1410.

HENSHAW, P. S., RILEY, E. F., and STAPLETON, G. E., *Radiology*, 1947, **49**, 349.

JORDAN, D. L., CLARK, J. W., and VOGEL, H. H., *Radiation Research*, 1956, **4**, 77.

KALLMAN, R. F., and KOHN, H. I., *Radiation Research*, 1955, **2**, 280.

KOHN, H. I., and KALLMAN, R. F., *Brit. J. Radiol.*, 1954, **27**, 586.

LEA, D. E., *Actions of Radiations on Living Cells*, 1946, Cambridge.

LORENZ, E., HESTON, W. E., ESCHENBRENNER, A. B., and DERINGER, M. K., *Radiology*, 1947, **49**, 274.

MOLE, R. H., *J. Nat. Cancer Institute*, 1955, **15**, 907.

MOLE, R. H., MUNSON, R. J., and NEARY, G. J., in *Radiobiology Symposium*, 1954, (ed. BACQ, Z. M., and ALEXANDER, P.), 1955, London.

SAMPFORD, M. R., *Biometrics*, 1952, **8**, 13 and 307.

STORER, J. B., and LANGHAM, W., Los Alamos Scientific Laboratory Report, 1953, LA-1630.

WORMAN, F. C. V., TURNEY, D. F., and LOTZ. V., Los Alamos Scientific Laboratory Report, 1954, LA-1641.

GENERAL SUMMARY AND CONCLUSIONS

THE experiment described here is believed to be unique in the sense that the continuous running of a nuclear reactor for several years was an integral part of a biological investigation. A nuclear reactor was used intermittently for short intense daily exposures by Henshaw *et al.* (1946, 1947) but the great advantage of using a reactor through the whole twenty-four hours was that the living conditions for the experimental animals could be made ideal. It was possible to use a nuclear reactor in this way only because of daily co-operation with physicists who appreciated that biological information was worth getting.

Thermal neutrons escaping from the nuclear reactor were used to make fast neutrons by fission in uranium slabs arranged in a horizontal plane just below the animals to be irradiated. A full description is given of the experimental arrangements including the methods of removing unwanted gamma rays and thermal neutrons and of dose control. Four different dose levels of fast neutrons from about one rad per day and downwards were obtained and one hundred mice were irradiated at each dose level till death. The mice lived permanently at the site of irradiation; there was no need for daily transfer of animals from living quarters to exposure cages with all the unwanted experimental variation which this involves. The irradiation was almost continuous: on an average 26 hours weekly were free from irradiation.

The doses of fast neutrons, gamma radiation and thermal neutrons were measured by the use of three chambers with differential sensitivities to the three kinds of radiation. A homogeneous chamber containing acetylene served as a fairly close approximation to tissue in its response to fast neutrons and gamma radiation. A second chamber of magnesium filled with argon responded to gamma radiation as would tissue but was insensitive to fast neutrons. Both of these chambers were insensitive to slow neutrons, which were measured by a third chamber containing boron trifluoride, which was relatively insensitive to fast neutrons and gamma radiation. Quite precise estimates of the separate effects of the three kinds of radiation in the three chambers were possible by making use of an approximate value for the energy of the fast neutrons (mean energy 0·7 MeV), and from this information the true tissue doses in rads could be obtained. The doses obtained in this way were confirmed by the use of a chamber the walls and gas filling of which approximated closely to soft tissue in their composition. The uncertainty in the estimate of fast neutron dose is about ten per cent, arising largely from uncertainty as to the energy expended in the formation of an ion pair by the slower-moving recoil atoms produced by the fast neutrons.

The effect of 0·54 rads weekly of fast neutrons on the life span of CBA mice was small and its statistical significance was uncertain. The higher dose of 6·4 rads weekly did not effect the white blood cell count but caused a marked drop in body weight and shortened life by one-third. After 2–5 months at 6·4 rads weekly, fertility in both males and females was seriously impaired. The reproductive function was found to be the most sensitive indicator of chronic radiation damage.

The majority of the mice, both irradiated and controls, died without the cause of death being discovered. Mammary tumours and malignant tumours of the nasopharynx, which normally occur rarely and late in life, were increased in frequency and also occurred earlier in CBA mice given 6·4 rads weekly of fast neutrons. Other killing tumours, which normally occur earlier in life, were not increased in frequency by the irradiation.

Additional information was obtained showing that experiments in which daily irradiation is given till the day of death may over-estimate the amount of radiation required to kill.

The interpretation of the results of chronic toxicological experiments such as these is discussed.

The relative biological efficiency of fast neutrons and ^{60}Co gamma radiation was determined for reduction in testis weight by exposures up to seven months, for impairment of male fertility by a nine weeks' exposure, for impairment of female fertility by irradiation for up to nine months, for reduction of the white blood cell count and of the weight of the spleen by irradiation for up to nine months. The values lay between 3 and 11. There were significant differences in the r.b.e. for testis weight reduction between genetically different mice, due mostly to quantitative differences in their response to gamma radiation. On the other hand the r.b.e. for damage to female fertility was apparently the same for the same three mouse strains, in spite of a fivefold difference in their intrinsic radiosensitivity. The r.b.e. for damage to the female gonad was consistently less than the r.b.e. for damage to the male gonad, and this could not be accounted for by differences in the actual dose received by organs at different depths below the surface of the animal. No evidence was obtained by us that the r.b.e. increased with the duration of exposure, i.e. with decrease in dose rate. A comparison of all available information on mortality of chronically irradiated mice suggested that the r.b.e. for this effect is likely to be about 10.

N*

Existing data for the r.b.e. for exposure to chronic irradiation were examined critically and it was shown that some methods of deriving the r.b.e. were inadmissible or open to serious possibilities of error. When recovery from radiation damage occurs only one method is permissible, the comparison of dose rates which produce the same degree of damage in the same time after the onset of irradiation.

GLOSSARY OF SYMBOLS

δ	density of the gas in an ionization chamber.
Δ	density of the wall of an ionization chamber.
ϵ	kinetic energy of a neutron or initial kinetic energy of an ionizing particle.
$^*\epsilon$	instantaneous kinetic energy of an ionizing particle.
ϵ_T	energy of $3kT/2$.
η	ionization efficiency of a particle relative to that of a similar particle of infinite energy.
θ	angle of scattering of a neutron in centre of mass coordinates.
κ	cross section per electron for pair production.
λ and μ	numerical constants which are measures of the dependence of $W(\epsilon)$ upon ϵ and of $^*W(^*v)$ upon $^*v$ respectively.
ρ	ratio of mass stopping powers of the wall and gas of an ionization chamber for the secondary particles traversing it.
σ_a	cross section per electron associated with energy absorption by Compton recoil electrons.
σ_g and σ_w	neutron scattering cross sections for atoms of the gas and wall of an ionization chamber.
$\sigma_i(\epsilon)$ and $\sigma_i(\theta, \epsilon)$	total and differential elastic scattering cross sections for neutrons of energy ϵ by atoms of type i.
$_a\sigma_i(\epsilon)$	absorption cross section for neutrons of energy ϵ by atoms of type i.
τ	photoelectric absorption cross section per electron.
A_i	atomic weight of an atom of type i.
a and b	internal and external radii of outer electrode of cylindrical (or spherical) ionization chamber.
$a_1, a_2 \ldots$	ionization rates (number of ions per unit mass of gas per unit time) in chambers 1, 2 ... exposed to gamma radiation at a dose rate of 1 r/hr.
$b_1, b_2 \ldots$	ionization rates in chambers 1, 2 ... exposed to fast neutrons at a dose rate of 1 rad/hr.
$c_1, c_2 \ldots$	ionization rates in chambers 1, 2 ... exposed to unit flux of slow neutrons.
$_\gamma D$ and $_n D$	dose rates of gamma radiation and fast neutrons respectively.
$d_1, d_2 \ldots$	gamma ray dose rates at chambers 1, 2 ... during calibration.
$_\gamma E_i$, $_n E_i$ and $_s E_i$	energy absorption in atoms of type i per unit mass of medium per unit time due to gamma radiation, fast neutrons and slow neutrons.
$E(\alpha)$ and $K(\alpha)$	complete elliptic integrals.
e	charge of the electron, or base of natural logarithms.
f_i	ratio of rate of decay of neutron induced radioactivity to its rate of production.
G	energy flux of gamma radiation.
$H_1, H_2 \ldots$	numerical factors relating ionization rate in chambers 1, 2 ... with reading of the current measuring instrument ($J_1 = M_1/H_1$, $J_2 = M_2/H_2 \ldots$).

h	Planck's constant.
${}_{\gamma}J$ and ${}_{n}J$	ionization per unit mass of gas per unit time due to gamma rays and fast neutrons respectively.
${}_{c}J_1$, ${}_{c}J_2$ ...	ionization rates in chambers 1, 2 ... during calibration with standard gamma ray source.
$j(\theta)$ and $\bar{j}$	number of ions produced by a neutron recoil ejected at the neutron scattering angle θ and the number averaged over all angles respectively.
$K_i(\epsilon)$	ratio of mean energy lost by a neutron of energy ϵ when elastically scattered by an atom i to that which would occur if the scattering were isotropic in centre of mass coordinates.
k	Boltzmann's constant.
l	average length of tracks of ionizing particles in the gas volume of an ionization chamber.
M_1, ${}_{c}M_1$	reading of the ionization current meter (in arbitrary units) in conjunction with chamber 1, reading during calibration of chamber 1.
m	exponent in the relation, range $\propto$ (energy) ^{m}, or mass per unit area of wall of ionization chamber.
N	flux of fast neutrons.
$N(\epsilon)\,d\epsilon$	flux of neutrons with energies between ϵ and $\epsilon+d\epsilon$.
$N(\nu)\,d\nu$	flux of photons with energies between $h\nu$ and $h(\nu+d\nu)$.
n_i	number of atoms of type i per unit mass of medium
p	partial pressure of one component in a mixture of gases.
$p_1, q_1, r_1; p_2, q_2, r_2; \ldots$	fractional losses in walls of chambers 1, 2, ... of gamma ray energy flux, fast neutron energy flux and slow neutron flux respectively.
Q and Q'	energy released when a neutron is captured by a single atomic nucleus and that released by a radioactive nucleus following neutron capture.
R and R'	ranges in the gas of an ionization chamber of recoils generated in the wall and gas respectively.
r	reflection coefficient for electrons at the inner surface of the wall of an ionization chamber.
S	flux of slow neutrons.
s_g and s_w	atomic (or electronic) stopping powers of gas and wall for neutron recoils (or secondary electrons) generated in the wall of an ionization chamber.
T	absolute temperature.
V	chamber voltage or chamber volume.
v and $^*v$	initial and instantaneous speeds of an ionizing particle.
v_0	speed of an electron in the first Bohn orbit of the hydrogen atom.
W_e, W_α ...	energy dissipation per ion pair produced in a gas by an electron, alpha particle ... .
$W(\epsilon)$ and $W(v)$	energy per ion pair for an ionizing particle of initial energy ϵ and initial speed v.
$^*W(^*\epsilon)$ and $^*W(^*v)$	instantaneous value of the energy per ion pair for a particle with energy $^*\epsilon$ and speed $^*v$.
$W(\infty)$	energy per ion pair for a particle as its energy tends to infinity.

INDEX

Printed in Great Britain by J. W. Arrowsmith Ltd., Bristol